Welcome to the ***"Snack Cookbook for Teens: Satisfy Your Snack Cravings with Fun and Easy Recipes With 115+ Recipes."***

Snacking is an essential part of a teen's day. Whether you're fueling up for a busy day at school, recharging after sports practice, or just hanging out with friends, the right snacks can make all the difference. This cookbook is designed to help you discover a wide variety of delicious, fun, and easy-to-make snacks that will satisfy your cravings and keep you energized throughout the day.

Why Snacking Matters

Snacks are more than just a quick bite between meals; they can provide essential nutrients, boost your energy levels, and help you maintain focus and concentration. For teens, who are constantly growing and on the go, having healthy and tasty snacks readily available is crucial. This cookbook aims to strike the perfect balance between nutrition and flavor, ensuring that every recipe is both enjoyable and beneficial for your body.

What You'll Find in This Cookbook

Inside, you'll find over 115 recipes that cater to all kinds of snack cravings. From sweet treats and savory bites to healthy options and indulgent delights, there's something for everyone. Each recipe is straightforward and easy to follow, making it perfect for both novice cooks and those with more kitchen experience.

Healthy and Fun

Eating well doesn't have to be boring. This cookbook includes a variety of recipes that are not only good for you but also fun to make and eat. You'll find recipes that use wholesome ingredients to create snacks that are as nutritious as they are tasty. Whether you're looking for a quick after-school bite or something to share with friends, these snacks will hit the spot.

Get Creative in the Kitchen

This cookbook encourages you to get creative and experiment with different flavors and ingredients. Feel free to tweak the recipes to suit your taste preferences or dietary needs. The kitchen is your playground, and these recipes are just the beginning of your culinary adventure.

Snack Time Made Easy

With simple instructions and easy-to-find ingredients, this cookbook makes snacking a breeze. Each recipe includes step-by-step directions, tips for success, and nutritional information to help you make informed choices. Whether you have a few minutes or a bit more time to spare, you'll find recipes that fit your schedule and satisfy your snack cravings.

Join the Snack Revolution

Get ready to transform the way you think about snacks. The "Snack Cookbook for Teens" is your ultimate guide to delicious, fun, and easy snacking. Dive into these recipes, explore new flavors, and enjoy the process of making and eating your snacks. Let's get snacking!

1. Greek Yogurt with Honey and Berries

Ingredient:

- 1 cup plain Greek yogurt
- 2 tbsp honey
- 1/2 cup mixed berries (such as blueberries, raspberries, blackberries)

Instructions:

1. Scoop the Greek yogurt into a bowl.

2. Drizzle the honey over the top of the yogurt.

3. Gently fold the honey into the yogurt until it is swirled throughout.

4. Top the yogurt with the mixed berries.

5. Serve immediately and enjoy!

This makes a delicious and healthy breakfast or snack. The creamy Greek yogurt paired with the sweetness of the honey and the freshness of the berries is a wonderful flavor combination. Feel free to adjust the amounts of honey or berries to your taste preferences.

2. Peanut Butter and Banana on Whole Grain Toast

Ingredient:

- 2 slices of whole grain bread
- 2 tablespoons of creamy peanut butter
- 1 ripe banana, sliced

Instructions:

1. Toast the whole grain bread until lightly golden brown.

2. Spread the peanut butter evenly over the toast slices.

3. Arrange the sliced banana on top of the peanut butter.

4. Serve immediately and enjoy!

This makes for a nutritious and satisfying breakfast or snack. The combination of the creamy peanut butter, sweet banana, and hearty whole grain bread provides a balance of protein, carbohydrates, and healthy fats to keep you feeling full and energized. Feel free to adjust the amounts of peanut butter and banana to your personal taste preferences.

3. Turkey and Cheese Roll•Ups

Ingredient:

- 8 slices deli turkey
- 4 slices cheddar cheese
- 2 tbsp cream cheese, softened
- 1 tbsp honey mustard
- 1 tsp dried parsley
- Salt and pepper to taste

Instructions:

1. Lay the turkey slices out flat on a clean surface.

2. In a small bowl, mix together the cream cheese, honey mustard, parsley, salt, and pepper until well combined.

3. Spread a thin layer of the cream cheese mixture evenly over each turkey slice.

4. Place a slice of cheddar cheese on top of the cream cheese on each turkey slice.

5. Tightly roll up each turkey slice, starting from the short end and rolling up into a spiral.

6. Secure the roll•ups with toothpicks if needed.

7. Refrigerate the roll•ups for at least 30 minutes to allow the cheese to set.

8. Remove the toothpicks and slice the roll•ups into 1•inch pieces before serving.

Enjoy these easy and flavorful turkey and cheese roll•ups as a quick snack or appetizer! The combination of the savory turkey, creamy cheese, and tangy honey mustard makes them a crowd•pleasing favorite.

8. Hummus with Carrot and Celery Sticks

Ingredient:

- 1 (15 oz) can chickpeas (garbanzo beans), drained and rinsed
- 2 tbsp tahini (sesame seed paste)
- 2 tbsp fresh lemon juice
- 1 garlic clove, minced
- 2 tbsp olive oil
- 1/4 tsp ground cumin
- 1/4 tsp salt
- 2•3 tbsp water, as needed
- 4•6 medium carrots, peeled and cut into sticks
- 4•6 celery stalks, cut into sticks

Instructions:

1. In a food processor or high•powered blender, combine the drained and rinsed chickpeas, tahini, lemon juice, garlic, olive oil, cumin, and salt. Blend until smooth, scraping down the sides as needed.

2. If the hummus is too thick, add 1•2 tablespoons of water and blend again until you reach your desired consistency.

3. Transfer the hummus to a serving bowl.

4. Arrange the carrot and celery sticks around the edge of the hummus bowl. Serve immediately or refrigerate until ready to enjoy.

The key components:

Hummus:
- Chickpeas provide protein, fiber, and complex carbs.
- Tahini adds creaminess and healthy fats.
- Lemon juice, garlic, and spices enhance the flavor.

Carrot and Celery Sticks:
- These fresh, crunchy veggies are perfect for dipping in the hummus.
- They add vitamins, minerals, and hydration.

This snack is a great balance of protein, healthy fats, complex carbs, and fiber. The hummus provides a creamy, savory dip while the carrot and celery sticks offer a refreshing crunch.

9. Low•Fat String Cheese

Ingredient:

- 1 gallon skim or low•fat milk
- 1/4 cup white vinegar or lemon juice
- 1/2 teaspoon salt

Equipment Needed:

- Large pot
- Cheesecloth or muslin
- Slotted spoon
- Knife or scissors

Instructions:

1. In a large pot, bring the milk to a gentle boil over medium heat, stirring frequently to prevent scorching.

2. Once the milk comes to a boil, remove the pot from the heat and stir in the vinegar or lemon juice. The milk should start to curdle and separate into curds and whey.

3. Allow the mixture to sit for 5•10 minutes, until the curds have fully formed and the whey is clear.

4. Using a slotted spoon, gently scoop the curds out of the pot and transfer them to a cheesecloth or muslin•lined colander. Allow the curds to drain for 5•10 minutes.

5. Transfer the drained curds to a clean work surface. Knead and stretch the curds with your hands until they become smooth and elastic, about 5•10 minutes.

6. Shape the stretched curds into string cheese sticks or logs. Sprinkle with salt and refrigerate until ready to use.

7. To serve, simply pull apart the string cheese into long, stringy pieces.

This homemade low•fat string cheese is a great healthy snack option. It's high in protein and low in fat and calories. Enjoy!

10. Almonds and Apple Slices

Ingredient:

- 1/4 cup raw, unsalted almonds
- 1 medium apple, cored and sliced

Instructions:

1. Arrange the apple slices on a plate or in a bowl.

2. Place the almonds next to the apple slices.

That's it! This makes a quick, easy, and nutritious snack.

The key components:

Almonds:
- Almonds are a great source of healthy fats, protein, fiber, and various vitamins and minerals.
- Choose raw, unsalted almonds for the most nutritional benefits.

Apples:
- Apples provide natural sweetness and crunch.
- They are high in fiber and antioxidants.

This combination of the crunchy, protein•rich almonds and the crisp, juicy apple slices makes for a satisfying and balanced snack. The flavors and textures complement each other nicely.

You can also try:
- Sprinkling a pinch of cinnamon over the apple slices
- Drizzling a small amount of honey or nut butter over the apples
- Substituting other nuts like walnuts or cashews

This simple snack is portable, easy to prepare, and provides a nice mix of nutrients to keep you feeling full and energized. Enjoy!

11. Turkey Jerky

Ingredient:

- 1 lb boneless, skinless turkey breast, thinly sliced
- 2 tbsp soy sauce
- 1 tbsp Worcestershire sauce
- 1 tsp smoked paprika
- 1 tsp garlic powder
- 1/2 tsp onion powder
- 1/2 tsp black pepper
- 1/4 tsp red pepper flakes (optional for spicy jerky)

Instructions:

1. In a large resealable bag or bowl, combine the soy sauce, Worcestershire sauce, smoked paprika, garlic powder, onion powder, black pepper, and red pepper flakes (if using). Add the turkey slices and toss to coat evenly.

2. Cover and marinate the turkey in the refrigerator for 2•4 hours, turning the bag occasionally to ensure even marinating.

3. Preheat your oven to 175°F (80°C). Line 2•3 baking sheets with parchment paper.

4. Remove the turkey slices from the marinade and arrange them in a single layer on the prepared baking sheets, making sure the slices are not touching.

5. Bake for 4•6 hours, flipping the jerky halfway through, until the turkey is dry and leathery. The exact time may vary depending on the thickness of the slices.

6. Allow the jerky to cool completely before storing. Store the turkey jerky in an airtight container at room temperature for up to 1 week.

Tips:
- Slice the turkey against the grain for a more tender jerky.
- Use a food dehydrator instead of the oven for a chewier texture.
- Experiment with different seasonings and marinades to create your own unique flavors.

Enjoy your homemade, protein•packed turkey jerky as a healthy snack!

12. Roasted Chickpeas

Ingredient:

- 1 (15 oz) can chickpeas (garbanzo beans), drained and rinsed
- 1 tbsp olive oil
- 1 tsp ground cumin
- 1 tsp paprika
- 1/2 tsp garlic powder
- 1/4 tsp salt
- 1/4 tsp black pepper

Instructions:

1. Preheat your oven to 400°F (200°C).

2. Drain and rinse the chickpeas, then pat them dry thoroughly with paper towels or a clean kitchen towel. This helps them get crispy.

3. In a medium bowl, toss the chickpeas with the olive oil, cumin, paprika, garlic powder, salt, and pepper until evenly coated.

4. Spread the seasoned chickpeas out in a single layer on a baking sheet lined with parchment paper.

5. Roast for 20•25 minutes, shaking the pan halfway, until the chickpeas are crispy and golden brown.

6. Remove from the oven and let cool for 5 minutes before serving.

The roasted chickpeas make a great crunchy, protein•packed snack on their own. You can also use them as a topping for salads, soups, or grain bowls.

Feel free to experiment with different spice blends too • try chili powder, cayenne, lemon pepper, or Italian seasoning for variety.

Enjoy your crispy, flavorful roasted chickpeas!

13. Low•Fat Cottage Cheese with Cucumber

Ingredient:

- 1 cup low•fat or non•fat cottage cheese
- 1/2 cucumber, diced
- 1 tbsp chopped fresh dill (or 1 tsp dried dill)
- 1/4 tsp salt
- 1/8 tsp black pepper

Instructions:

1. In a small bowl, combine the cottage cheese, diced cucumber, dill, salt, and black pepper. Stir gently to mix.

2. Serve immediately or refrigerate until ready to eat.

That's it! This makes a quick, easy, and nutritious snack or light meal.

The key components:

Cottage Cheese:
- Look for low•fat or non•fat cottage cheese to keep the calories and fat low.
- Cottage cheese is high in protein and calcium.

Cucumber:
- Cucumber adds a refreshing crunch and hydration.
- It's low in calories and high in vitamins and minerals.

Dill:
- Fresh dill adds a bright, herbal flavor.
- Dried dill works well too if you don't have fresh.

Salt and Pepper:
- Season to taste to bring out the flavors.

You can also try adding other fresh herbs, a squeeze of lemon juice, or a sprinkle of red pepper flakes for extra flavor.

This makes a great snack or light lunch. The cottage cheese provides protein while the cucumber keeps it light and hydrating. Enjoy!

14. Greek Yogurt with a Sprinkle of Granola

Ingredient:

- 1 cup plain Greek yogurt
- 2•3 tablespoons granola

Instructions:

1. Scoop the Greek yogurt into a bowl or serving dish.

2. Sprinkle the granola evenly over the top of the yogurt.

That's it! This healthy snack or breakfast is ready to enjoy.

The key things to note:

Greek Yogurt:
- Greek yogurt is thicker, creamier, and higher in protein than regular yogurt. Look for plain, unsweetened varieties.

Granola:
- Choose a granola that is low in added sugars. Look for ones made with whole grains, nuts, seeds, and minimal sweeteners.

You can also customize this further by adding:
- Fresh fruit like berries, sliced banana, or diced apple
- A drizzle of honey or maple syrup
- A sprinkle of cinnamon or nutmeg
- Chopped nuts or seeds

The combination of the tangy Greek yogurt and the crunchy, lightly sweet granola makes for a delicious and nutritious snack or breakfast. It's quick, easy, and satisfying.

15. Chia Seed Pudding with Vanilla Almond Milk

Ingredient:

- 1/4 cup chia seeds
- 1 cup unsweetened vanilla almond milk
- 1 tbsp maple syrup (or honey)
- 1/2 tsp vanilla extract
- Pinch of cinnamon (optional)
- Fresh fruit for topping (such as berries, sliced banana, etc.)

Instructions:

1. In a medium bowl, whisk together the chia seeds, almond milk, maple syrup, and vanilla extract until well combined.

2. Cover the bowl and refrigerate for at least 2 hours, or overnight, stirring occasionally, until the mixture has thickened to a pudding•like consistency.

3. When ready to serve, give the chia pudding a final stir. Spoon it into serving bowls or jars.

4. Top the chia pudding with your choice of fresh fruit. Optionally, sprinkle a pinch of cinnamon over the top.

That's it! This chia seed pudding is a nutritious and delicious snack or breakfast.

The key components:

Chia Seeds:
- Chia seeds are packed with fiber, protein, omega•3s, and other beneficial nutrients.
- They thicken the pudding and give it a satisfying, creamy texture.

Vanilla Almond Milk:
- Unsweetened vanilla almond milk provides creaminess and natural sweetness.
- It's a dairy•free, low•calorie alternative to regular milk.

Maple Syrup (or Honey):
- A small amount of maple syrup or honey adds just the right amount of sweetness.

Fresh Fruit:
- Topping the pudding with fresh fruit like berries, banana, or mango adds natural sweetness and extra nutrients

16. Protein Bars with Low Sugar

Ingredient:

- 1 cup rolled oats
- 1/2 cup unsweetened shredded coconut
- 1/2 cup creamy peanut butter (or other nut butter)
- 1/4 cup honey or maple syrup
- 1 scoop (about 30g) vanilla protein powder
- 1/4 cup unsweetened almond milk
- 1/4 tsp sea salt

Instructions:

1. Line an 8x8 inch baking pan with parchment paper and set aside.

2. In a large bowl, mix together the rolled oats, shredded coconut, protein powder, and salt.

3. In a small saucepan, heat the peanut butter and honey/maple syrup over low heat, stirring constantly, until smooth and combined.

4. Pour the warm peanut butter mixture into the dry ingredients and stir until well coated.

5. Stir in the almond milk until a thick, sticky dough forms.

6. Transfer the dough to the prepared baking pan and press it down evenly with your hands or a spatula.

7. Refrigerate for at least 2 hours, or until firm.

8. Remove the bars from the pan using the parchment paper and cut into 8•10 bars. Store the protein bars in an airtight container in the refrigerator for up to 1 week.

The key features:
Low•Sugar:
- Using honey or maple syrup instead of refined sugar keeps the added sugar content low.

Protein•Packed:
- The protein powder boosts the protein content to help keep you full and satisfied.

Healthy Fats:
- The nut butter and coconut provide heart•healthy fats.

17. Tuna Salad Lettuce Wraps

Ingredient:

- 1 (5 oz) can tuna, drained and flaked
- 2 tbsp plain Greek yogurt
- 1 tbsp diced celery
- 1 tbsp diced red onion
- 1 tsp Dijon mustard
- 1 tsp lemon juice
- Salt and pepper to taste
- 4•6 large lettuce leaves (such as romaine or butter lettuce)

Instructions:

1. In a small bowl, mix together the drained tuna, Greek yogurt, celery, red onion, Dijon mustard, and lemon juice. Season with salt and pepper to taste.

2. Lay the lettuce leaves flat on a plate or cutting board.

3. Scoop a portion of the tuna salad mixture onto the center of each lettuce leaf. Wrap the lettuce around the tuna salad, burrito•style, and enjoy.

The key components:

Tuna:
- Canned tuna is a great source of lean protein.
- Choose tuna packed in water rather than oil for a lower•fat option.

Greek Yogurt:
- Using Greek yogurt instead of mayo keeps the tuna salad creamy but lower in fat and calories.

Veggies:
- The celery and onion add a nice crunch and flavor.

Lettuce Wraps:
- Lettuce leaves make a refreshing, low•carb alternative to bread or crackers.

This tuna salad lettuce wrap is a light, healthy, and portable snack or lunch. The tuna provides protein to keep you full, while the crunchy veggies and cool lettuce make it a satisfying and nutritious option

18. Sliced Bell Peppers with Hummus

Ingredient:

• 1 medium bell pepper (any color), sliced into strips
• 1/4 cup prepared hummus

Instructions:

1. Wash the bell pepper and slice it into long, thin strips.

2. Arrange the bell pepper strips on a plate or in a bowl.

3. Scoop the hummus into a small dish or ramekin and place it next to the bell pepper strips.

That's it! This makes a quick, easy, and nutritious snack.

The key components:

Bell Peppers:
• Bell peppers are crunchy, juicy, and packed with vitamins, minerals, and antioxidants.
• The vibrant colors add visual appeal.

Hummus:
• Hummus is a creamy, protein•rich dip made from chickpeas, tahini, olive oil, and spices.
• It provides healthy fats, fiber, and plant•based protein.

This combination of fresh, crisp bell pepper strips and creamy, flavorful hummus makes for a satisfying and balanced snack. The peppers provide a nice crunch and hydration, while the hummus adds protein and healthy fats to keep you feeling full.

You can use any color of bell pepper • red, yellow, orange, or green. The flavors will vary slightly, but they all work great with the hummus.

Feel free to experiment with different hummus flavors as well, such as roasted red pepper, garlic, or Mediterranean•style. Enjoy this simple, nutritious snack!

19. Cottage Cheese with Strawberries

Ingredient:

- 1 cup low•fat or non•fat cottage cheese
- 1 cup fresh strawberries, sliced
- 1 tsp honey (optional)

Instructions:

1. In a small bowl, combine the cottage cheese and sliced strawberries.

2. If desired, drizzle the honey over the top and gently stir to combine.

That's it! This makes a quick, easy, and nutritious snack or light breakfast.

The key components:

Cottage Cheese:
- Cottage cheese is high in protein and low in fat, making it a great healthy choice.
- Look for low•fat or non•fat varieties to keep the calorie and fat content down.

Strawberries:
- Fresh, juicy strawberries add natural sweetness and a boost of vitamin C.
- Strawberries also provide fiber and antioxidants.

Honey (optional):
- A small drizzle of honey can enhance the sweetness if desired, but it's optional.

This simple combination of creamy cottage cheese and sweet, fresh strawberries makes for a refreshing and satisfying snack. The protein from the cottage cheese helps keep you feeling full and satisfied.

You can also try adding other fresh fruit like blueberries, raspberries, or diced peaches for variety. Enjoy this healthy and delicious cottage cheese and strawberry treat!

20. Protein-Packed Pancakes

Ingredient:

- 1 cup rolled oats
- 1/2 cup plain Greek yogurt
- 2 large eggs
- 1 scoop (about 30g) vanilla protein powder
- 1 tsp baking powder
- 1/4 tsp salt
- 1/4 cup unsweetened almond milk (or milk of your choice)
- 1 tsp vanilla extract
- Toppings (such as fresh berries, sliced banana, maple syrup, etc.)

Instructions:

1. In a blender or food processor, blend the rolled oats until they reach a flour•like consistency.

2. Add the Greek yogurt, eggs, protein powder, baking powder, salt, almond milk, and vanilla extract. Blend until a smooth batter forms.

3. Heat a non•stick skillet or griddle over medium heat. Lightly grease the surface with a small amount of oil or non•stick cooking spray.

4. Scoop the batter onto the hot surface, using about 1/4 cup per pancake. Cook for 2•3 minutes per side, or until golden brown. Serve the protein pancakes warm, topped with your desired toppings.

The key components:

Oats: Blending the oats into a flour provides complex carbs and fiber.

Greek Yogurt: The yogurt adds protein, creaminess, and moisture to the pancakes.

Protein Powder: The vanilla protein powder boosts the overall protein content.

Eggs: Eggs contribute more protein and help bind the pancake batter.

These protein•packed pancakes are a nutritious and satisfying breakfast or snack. The combination of oats, protein, and healthy fats will help keep you feeling full and energized.

21. Mini Egg Muffins with Vegetables

Ingredient:

- 6 large eggs
- 1/4 cup diced bell pepper
- 1/4 cup diced onion
- 1/4 cup diced spinach or kale
- 2 tbsp unsweetened almond milk
- 1/4 tsp salt
- 1/8 tsp black pepper

Instructions:

1. Preheat your oven to 350°F (175°C). Grease a 12•cup mini muffin tin with non•stick cooking spray.

2. In a medium bowl, whisk the eggs together with the almond milk, salt, and pepper until well combined.

3. Stir in the diced bell pepper, onion, and spinach/kale until evenly distributed.

4. Carefully pour the egg mixture into the prepared muffin cups, filling each one about 3/4 full.

5. Bake for 18•22 minutes, until the egg muffins are set and lightly golden brown on top. Remove the muffin tin from the oven and let the egg muffins cool in the tin for 5 minutes. Use a fork or spoon to gently remove the egg muffins from the tin. Serve warm.

The key components:

Eggs: Eggs provide high•quality protein to keep you feeling full.

Vegetables: The bell pepper, onion, and spinach/kale add fiber, vitamins, and minerals.

Almond Milk: Using unsweetened almond milk keeps the muffins low in calories and fat.

These mini egg muffins make a great healthy breakfast, snack, or on•the•go option. The vegetables add flavor and nutrition, while the small size makes them easy to grab and go.

Feel free to experiment with different veggie combinations, such as mushrooms, tomatoes, or broccoli. You can also add a sprinkle of cheese on top if desired. Enjoy these nutritious egg muffins!

22. Chicken Salad on Whole Wheat Crackers

Ingredient:

- 2 cups cooked, shredded chicken breast
- 1/4 cup plain Greek yogurt
- 1 tbsp Dijon mustard
- 1 tbsp lemon juice
- 1/4 cup diced celery
- 2 tbsp diced red onion
- 1 tbsp chopped fresh parsley
- Salt and pepper to taste
- 12•16 whole wheat crackers

Instructions:

1. In a medium bowl, mix together the shredded chicken, Greek yogurt, Dijon mustard, lemon juice, celery, red onion, and parsley. Season with salt and pepper to taste.

2. Scoop a spoonful of the chicken salad mixture onto each whole wheat cracker.

3. Serve the chicken salad crackers immediately.

The key components:

Chicken Salad:
- Using cooked, shredded chicken breast keeps the protein content high.
- The Greek yogurt provides creaminess while keeping the fat and calories low.
- The Dijon mustard, lemon juice, celery, onion, and parsley add flavor and crunch.

Whole Wheat Crackers:
- Whole wheat crackers are a nutritious, high•fiber base for the chicken salad.
- Look for crackers with minimal added sugars or oils.

This chicken salad on whole wheat crackers makes for a quick, easy, and healthy snack or light meal. The protein•rich chicken paired with the fiber•filled crackers creates a satisfying combination.

You can also serve the chicken salad on top of mixed greens, stuffed into celery sticks, or scooped onto sliced cucumber rounds for additional veggie servings.

Enjoy this simple and delicious chicken salad cracker snack!

23. Pumpkin Seeds

Ingredient:

- 1 cup raw pumpkin seeds (also called pepitas)
- 1 tbsp olive oil
- 1 tsp salt (or to taste)
- Optional seasonings: garlic powder, onion powder, chili powder, cumin, etc.

Instructions:

1. Preheat your oven to 325°F (165°C).

2. Rinse the pumpkin seeds under cold water to remove any pulp or strings. Pat them dry completely with paper towels.

3. In a small bowl, toss the clean, dry pumpkin seeds with the olive oil and salt (and any other desired seasonings).

4. Spread the seasoned pumpkin seeds in a single layer on a baking sheet lined with parchment paper.

5. Roast for 15•20 minutes, stirring halfway, until the seeds are lightly golden brown and crispy.

6. Remove the roasted pumpkin seeds from the oven and let them cool completely before serving.

That's it! These roasted pumpkin seeds make a delicious, crunchy, and nutritious snack.

Some tips:
- For best results, make sure the seeds are completely dry before roasting.
- Adjust the roasting time as needed, keeping an eye on them to prevent burning.
- Store the cooled roasted seeds in an airtight container for up to 1 week.

Pumpkin seeds are packed with healthy fats, protein, fiber, vitamins, and minerals. They make a great portable snack or topping for salads, yogurt, oatmeal, and more. Enjoy!

24. Baked Tofu Bites

Ingredient:

- 1 block (14 oz) extra•firm tofu, pressed and cut into 1•inch cubes
- 2 tbsp low•sodium soy sauce or tamari
- 1 tbsp maple syrup
- 1 tsp sesame oil
- 1 tsp garlic powder
- 1/2 tsp ground ginger
- 1/4 tsp red pepper flakes (optional for spicy tofu)

Instructions:

1. Preheat your oven to 400°F (200°C). Line a baking sheet with parchment paper.

2. In a medium bowl, whisk together the soy sauce, maple syrup, sesame oil, garlic powder, ginger, and red pepper flakes (if using).

3. Add the pressed and cubed tofu to the bowl and gently toss to coat the tofu pieces evenly with the marinade.

4. Arrange the marinated tofu cubes in a single layer on the prepared baking sheet.

5. Bake for 20•25 minutes, flipping the tofu pieces halfway, until they are golden brown and crispy on the outside. Remove the baked tofu bites from the oven and let them cool slightly before serving.

The key components:

Tofu:
- Extra•firm tofu provides a meaty texture and plant•based protein.
- Pressing the tofu helps remove excess moisture for better baking.

Soy Sauce/Tamari: The soy sauce or tamari adds a savory, umami flavor.

Maple Syrup: A touch of maple syrup balances the saltiness and adds a subtle sweetness.

Spices: The garlic, ginger, and optional red pepper flakes provide aromatic seasoning.

These baked tofu bites make a great protein•packed snack or addition to salads, bowls, and stir•fries. The crispy exterior and flavorful marinade make them irresistible.

25. Avocado and Tuna Salad

Ingredient:

- 1 (5 oz) can tuna, drained
- 1 ripe avocado, diced
- 2 tbsp plain Greek yogurt
- 1 tbsp lemon juice
- 1 tbsp diced red onion
- 1 tbsp diced celery
- 1 tsp Dijon mustard
- Salt and pepper to taste

Instructions:

1. In a medium bowl, gently mix together the drained tuna, diced avocado, Greek yogurt, lemon juice, red onion, celery, and Dijon mustard.

2. Season the salad with salt and pepper to taste.

3. Serve the avocado tuna salad on its own, on top of mixed greens, or with whole grain crackers or slices of cucumber.

The key components:

Tuna:
- Canned tuna is a lean protein that provides omega•3 fatty acids.
- Choose tuna packed in water rather than oil for a lower•fat option.

Avocado:
- Avocado adds healthy fats, fiber, and a creamy texture to the salad.
- It also provides vitamins, minerals, and antioxidants.

Greek Yogurt:
- Using Greek yogurt instead of mayonnaise keeps the salad lower in calories and fat.
- It adds creaminess and a boost of protein.

Vegetables:
- The red onion and celery provide crunch and flavor.

This avocado and tuna salad is a nutritious and delicious option for a light lunch or snack. The healthy fats from the avocado and omega•3s from the tuna make it a filling and satisfying choice.

26. Quinoa Salad with Veggies

Ingredient:

- 1 cup cooked quinoa, cooled
- 1/2 cup diced cucumber
- 1/2 cup diced cherry tomatoes
- 1/4 cup diced red onion
- 1/4 cup diced bell pepper
- 2 tbsp chopped fresh parsley
- 2 tbsp olive oil
- 1 tbsp lemon juice
- 1 tsp Dijon mustard
- 1/4 tsp salt
- 1/8 tsp black pepper

Instructions:

1. In a large bowl, combine the cooked and cooled quinoa, diced cucumber, tomatoes, red onion, bell pepper, and chopped parsley.

2. In a small bowl, whisk together the olive oil, lemon juice, Dijon mustard, salt, and black pepper.

3. Pour the dressing over the quinoa and vegetable mixture and toss gently to coat everything evenly. Serve the quinoa salad chilled or at room temperature.

The key components:

Quinoa:
- Quinoa is a nutrient•dense, gluten•free grain that provides protein, fiber, and complex carbs.

Fresh Vegetables:
- The cucumber, tomatoes, onion, and bell pepper add crunch, color, and a variety of vitamins and minerals.

Olive Oil and Lemon Dressing:
- The simple olive oil and lemon juice dressing adds flavor and healthy fats.
- The Dijon mustard helps emulsify the dressing.

This quinoa salad is a great make•ahead option for a healthy lunch or side dish. The combination of the fluffy quinoa, crisp veggies, and tangy dressing makes it a refreshing and satisfying choice.

27. Protein Balls with Oats and Peanut Butter

Ingredient:

- 1 cup old•fashioned rolled oats
- 1/2 cup creamy peanut butter
- 1/4 cup honey
- 1 scoop (about 30g) vanilla protein powder
- 2 tbsp ground flaxseed
- 1 tbsp chia seeds
- 1/4 tsp salt

Instructions:

1. In a medium bowl, mix together the rolled oats, peanut butter, honey, protein powder, flaxseed, chia seeds, and salt until well combined.

2. Using a tablespoon or small cookie scoop, form the mixture into small balls, about 1•inch in size.

3. Place the protein balls on a parchment•lined baking sheet or plate.

4. Refrigerate the protein balls for at least 30 minutes to allow them to firm up.

5. Store the protein balls in an airtight container in the refrigerator for up to 1 week.

The key components:

Oats: Rolled oats provide complex carbs, fiber, and texture.

Peanut Butter: Creamy peanut butter adds healthy fats and protein.

Protein Powder: The vanilla protein powder boosts the overall protein content.

Honey: Honey acts as a natural sweetener and binder.

Flaxseed and Chia Seeds: These add extra fiber, protein, and omega•3 fatty acids.

These protein balls make a great healthy snack or pre/post•workout treat. The combination of oats, peanut butter, and protein powder keeps you feeling full and satisfied.

Feel free to experiment with different nut butters, protein powder flavors, or add•ins like chocolate chips, coconut, or dried fruit. Enjoy these easy and nutritious protein balls!

28. Low•Fat Mozzarella Cheese Sticks

Ingredient:

• 8 oz part•skim mozzarella cheese, cut into 1/2•inch thick sticks
• 1/4 cup whole wheat breadcrumbs
• 1 tbsp grated Parmesan cheese
• 1 tsp dried oregano
• 1/4 tsp garlic powder
• 1 large egg, beaten
• Marinara sauce, for dipping (optional)

Instructions:

1. Preheat your oven to 400°F (200°C). Line a baking sheet with parchment paper.

2. In a shallow bowl, mix together the breadcrumbs, Parmesan cheese, oregano, and garlic powder.

3. Dip each mozzarella cheese stick first into the beaten egg, then roll it in the breadcrumb mixture, pressing gently to help it adhere.

4. Arrange the breaded cheese sticks on the prepared baking sheet.

5. Bake for 8•10 minutes, flipping halfway, until the cheese sticks are golden brown.

6. Serve the low•fat mozzarella cheese sticks warm, with marinara sauce for dipping if desired.

The key components:

Part•Skim Mozzarella: Using part•skim mozzarella keeps the cheese sticks lower in fat and calories.

Whole Wheat Breadcrumbs: Whole wheat breadcrumbs provide a crunchy coating with added fiber.

Parmesan Cheese: A small amount of Parmesan adds extra flavor and a touch of saltiness.

These baked, low•fat mozzarella cheese sticks are a healthier alternative to the traditional deep•fried version. They still have a crispy, crunchy exterior and a melty, cheesy interior, but with fewer calories and less fat.

29. Cottage Cheese with Blueberries

Ingredient:

- 1 cup low•fat or non•fat cottage cheese
- 1/2 cup fresh blueberries
- 1 tsp honey (optional)

Instructions:

1. In a small bowl, combine the cottage cheese and fresh blueberries.

2. If desired, drizzle the honey over the top and gently stir to combine.

That's it! This makes a quick, easy, and nutritious snack or light breakfast.

The key components:

Cottage Cheese:
- Cottage cheese is high in protein and low in fat, making it a great healthy choice.
- Look for low•fat or non•fat varieties to keep the calorie and fat content down.

Blueberries:
- Fresh blueberries add natural sweetness, fiber, and a boost of antioxidants.

Honey (optional):
- A small drizzle of honey can enhance the sweetness if desired, but it's optional.

This simple combination of creamy cottage cheese and juicy blueberries makes for a refreshing and satisfying snack or light meal. The protein from the cottage cheese helps keep you feeling full and satisfied.

You can also try adding other fresh fruit like raspberries, blackberries, or diced peaches for variety. Enjoy this healthy and delicious cottage cheese and blueberry treat!

30. Smoothie Bowl with Greek Yogurt and Fruit

Ingredient:

- 1 cup plain Greek yogurt
- 1 cup frozen mixed berries (such as blueberries, raspberries, and blackberries)
- 1/2 banana, frozen
- 1/2 cup unsweetened almond milk
- 1 tbsp honey (optional)
- Toppings: sliced banana, fresh berries, granola, chia seeds, etc.

Instructions:

1. In a high•powered blender, combine the Greek yogurt, frozen berries, frozen banana, and almond milk. Blend until smooth and creamy.

2. If desired, add the honey and blend again briefly to incorporate.

3. Pour the smoothie mixture into a bowl.

4. Top the smoothie bowl with your desired toppings, such as sliced banana, fresh berries, granola, chia seeds, or a drizzle of honey.

The key components:

Greek Yogurt:
- Greek yogurt provides a thick, creamy base that is high in protein.
- It adds creaminess and richness to the smoothie bowl.

Frozen Fruit:
- Using frozen berries and banana creates a cold, slushy texture.
- The fruit provides natural sweetness, fiber, and antioxidants.

Almond Milk:
- Unsweetened almond milk keeps the smoothie bowl light and low in calories.
- It helps blend the ingredients together smoothly.

Toppings:
- The toppings add texture, flavor, and extra nutrition.
- Fresh fruit, granola, and seeds make it a more substantial and satisfying meal or snack.

This smoothie bowl is a nutritious and delicious way to start your day or enjoy as a healthy snack. The combination of protein•rich Greek yogurt, antioxidant•packed fruit, and crunchy toppings makes it a well•balanced and satisfying option.

31. Turkey and Avocado on Whole Grain Crackers

Ingredient:

- 4•6 whole grain crackers
- 2•3 slices of deli turkey
- 1/2 avocado, sliced
- Salt and pepper to taste

Instructions:

1. Arrange the whole grain crackers on a plate or serving tray.

2. Top each cracker with a slice or two of deli turkey.

3. Place a few slices of avocado on top of the turkey.

4. Season with a pinch of salt and freshly ground black pepper.

That's it! This makes for a quick, healthy, and tasty snack or light meal. The combination of the savory turkey, creamy avocado, and crunchy whole grain crackers is really delicious. Feel free to adjust the amounts of each ingredient to your personal preference.

32. Protein Muffins with Banana and Oats

Ingredient:

- 1 cup mashed ripe banana (about 2 medium bananas)
- 1/2 cup unsweetened applesauce
- 1/4 cup honey or maple syrup
- 2 large eggs
- 1 scoop (about 30g) vanilla protein powder
- 1 cup rolled oats
- 1/2 cup whole wheat flour
- 1 tsp baking powder
- 1/2 tsp baking soda
- 1/4 tsp salt

Instructions:

1. Preheat your oven to 350°F (175°C). Grease a 12•cup muffin tin or line with paper liners.

2. In a large bowl, mash the ripe bananas. Stir in the applesauce, honey/maple syrup, and eggs until well combined.

3. In a separate bowl, mix together the protein powder, rolled oats, whole wheat flour, baking powder, baking soda, and salt.

4. Fold the dry ingredients into the wet ingredients until just combined, being careful not to overmix.

5. Divide the batter evenly among the prepared muffin cups, filling them about 3/4 full.

6. Bake for 18•22 minutes, until a toothpick inserted in the center comes out clean.

7. Allow the muffins to cool in the tin for 5 minutes before transferring to a wire rack.

These protein•packed banana oat muffins make a great healthy breakfast, snack, or on•the•go option. The combination of protein, complex carbs, and natural sweetness from the banana keeps you feeling full and satisfied.

Feel free to experiment with different protein powder flavors or add•ins like nuts, seeds, or dried fruit. Enjoy these nutritious and delicious protein muffins!

33. Spicy Roasted Edamame

Ingredient:

- 1 lb fresh edamame in the pod
- 2 tbsp olive oil
- 1 tsp chili powder
- 1/2 tsp garlic powder
- 1/4 tsp cayenne pepper (or to taste)
- 1/2 tsp salt

Instructions:

1. Preheat your oven to 400°F (200°C).

2. Rinse the edamame pods under cold water and pat them dry with paper towels.

3. In a large bowl, toss the edamame pods with the olive oil, chili powder, garlic powder, cayenne pepper, and salt until evenly coated.

4. Spread the seasoned edamame in a single layer on a large baking sheet lined with parchment paper.

5. Roast in the preheated oven for 12•15 minutes, stirring halfway, until the edamame are lightly browned and crispy.

6. Remove from the oven and let cool for 5 minutes before serving.

7. Serve the spicy roasted edamame warm, either in the pods or shelled. They make a great healthy snack or appetizer.

Enjoy the bold, spicy flavor of these roasted edamame! Adjust the amount of cayenne pepper to your desired level of heat.

34. Chia Pudding with Fresh Fruit

Ingredient:

- 1/4 cup chia seeds
- 1 cup unsweetened almond milk
- 1 tbsp maple syrup or honey (optional)
- 1 tsp vanilla extract
- 1 cup mixed fresh fruit (such as berries, diced mango, kiwi, etc.)

Instructions:

1. In a medium bowl, whisk together the chia seeds, almond milk, maple syrup/honey (if using), and vanilla extract until well combined.

2. Cover the bowl and refrigerate for at least 2 hours, or overnight, stirring occasionally, until the mixture has thickened to a pudding•like consistency.

3. When ready to serve, give the chia pudding a final stir. Divide the pudding into serving bowls or jars. Top each portion of chia pudding with the fresh mixed fruit.

That's it! This chia pudding with fresh fruit makes a delicious and nutritious snack or breakfast.

The key components:

Chia Seeds:
- Chia seeds are packed with fiber, protein, omega•3s, and other beneficial nutrients.
- They thicken the pudding and give it a satisfying, creamy texture.

Almond Milk:
- Unsweetened almond milk provides creaminess and a mild flavor.
- It's a dairy•free, low•calorie alternative to regular milk.

Maple Syrup or Honey (optional):
- A small amount of sweetener can be added if desired, but it's optional.

Fresh Fruit:
- Topping the chia pudding with a variety of fresh, seasonal fruit adds natural sweetness, fiber, and vitamins.

This chia pudding with fresh fruit is easy to make, full of nutrition, and can be enjoyed as a healthy snack, breakfast, or dessert. Feel free to adjust the sweetener to your taste preference. Enjoy!

35. Veggie Sticks with Greek Yogurt Dip

Ingredient:

Veggie Sticks:
- 1 carrot, peeled and cut into sticks
- 1 cucumber, cut into sticks
- 1 bell pepper, cut into sticks
- 1 celery stalk, cut into sticks

Greek Yogurt Dip:
- 1 cup plain Greek yogurt
- 2 tbsp fresh dill, chopped
- 1 tbsp lemon juice
- 1 garlic clove, minced
- 1/4 tsp salt
- 1/4 tsp black pepper

Instructions:

1. Prepare the veggie sticks by washing, peeling (if needed), and cutting the carrots, cucumber, bell pepper, and celery into long, thin sticks.

2. In a small bowl, mix together all the ingredients for the Greek yogurt dip • the yogurt, dill, lemon juice, garlic, salt, and pepper. Stir until well combined.

3. Arrange the veggie sticks on a platter or plate.

4. Serve the Greek yogurt dip alongside the veggie sticks for dipping.

That's it! This makes for a simple, healthy, and delicious snack or appetizer.

The key benefits:
- Vegetables provide fiber, vitamins, and minerals.
- Greek yogurt is high in protein and probiotics.
- The dill and lemon add fresh, zesty flavors to the dip.

You can customize this recipe by using different types of vegetables, such as broccoli florets, cherry tomatoes, or snow pea pods. You can also experiment with other herb and spice combinations in the dip.

Enjoy this nutritious and satisfying veggie and dip snack!

36. Protein•Packed Granola Bars

Ingredient:

- 2 cups old•fashioned oats
- 1/2 cup unsweetened shredded coconut
- 1/2 cup chopped nuts (such as almonds, walnuts, or pecans)
- 1/4 cup ground flaxseed
- 1/4 cup chia seeds
- 1/4 cup honey
- 1/4 cup creamy peanut butter (or other nut butter)
- 1 scoop (about 30g) vanilla protein powder
- 1 tsp vanilla extract
- 1/4 tsp salt

Instructions:

1. Preheat your oven to 325°F (165°C). Line an 8x8 inch baking pan with parchment paper, leaving some overhang on the sides for easy removal.

2. In a large bowl, combine the oats, shredded coconut, chopped nuts, flaxseed, and chia seeds. Mix well.

3. In a separate bowl, whisk together the honey, peanut butter, protein powder, vanilla extract, and salt until smooth.

4. Pour the wet ingredients into the dry ingredients and stir until everything is well combined.

5. Press the granola bar mixture firmly into the prepared baking pan, using your hands or the back of a spoon to compact it.

6. Bake for 20•25 minutes, until the edges are lightly golden brown.

7. Allow the granola bars to cool completely in the pan, then use the parchment paper to lift them out. Cut into 8•10 bars.

8. Store the granola bars in an airtight container at room temperature for up to 1 week, or in the refrigerator for up to 2 weeks.

These protein•packed granola bars are a great healthy snack or on•the•go breakfast option. The combination of oats, nuts, seeds, and protein powder makes them filling and nutritious.

37. Peanut Butter on Apple Slices

Ingredient:

- 1 apple, cored and sliced into wedges
- 2•3 tablespoons creamy peanut butter

Instructions:

1. Wash and core the apple. Slice it into wedges or thin slices.

2. Spread a small amount of peanut butter, about 1/2 to 1 teaspoon, onto each apple slice.

3. Arrange the peanut butter•topped apple slices on a plate or platter.

That's it! This makes for a quick, easy, and healthy snack.

The key benefits of this recipe:

- Apples provide fiber, vitamins, and antioxidants.
- Peanut butter is a good source of protein and healthy fats.
- It's a simple, no•cook snack that's satisfying and nutritious.

You can use any type of apple you prefer, such as Gala, Fuji, or Honeycrisp. For variety, you can also try using different nut butters like almond butter or cashew butter.

If desired, you can sprinkle a pinch of cinnamon over the peanut butter•topped apple slices for an extra flavor boost.

This snack is perfect for a quick pick•me•up, a healthy after•school treat, or even a light dessert. Enjoy!

38. Turkey Slices with Dijon Mustard

Ingredient:

- 4•6 slices of deli turkey
- 1•2 tbsp Dijon mustard
- Optional toppings: lettuce, tomato, onion, cheese

Instructions:

1. Lay the turkey slices out on a plate or cutting board.

2. Spread a thin layer of Dijon mustard over the top of each turkey slice, using about 1/2 to 1 teaspoon per slice.

3. If using any optional toppings, layer them over the mustard•coated turkey slices.

4. You can serve the turkey slices as is, or you can roll them up into mini wraps or sandwiches.

That's it! This makes for a quick, easy, and flavorful snack or light meal.

The key benefits of this recipe:

- Turkey is a lean protein that is high in nutrients.
- Dijon mustard adds a zesty, tangy flavor.
- The optional toppings can provide extra nutrients and crunch.

You can customize this recipe by using different types of mustard (e.g. honey mustard, spicy brown mustard), adding cheese, or using different vegetable toppings. It's a versatile and healthy option.

39. Baked Zucchini Chips with Greek Yogurt Dip

Ingredient:

Zucchini Chips:
- 2 medium zucchinis, sliced into 1/4•inch thick rounds
- 1 tbsp olive oil
- 1 tsp garlic powder
- 1 tsp paprika
- 1/2 tsp salt
- 1/4 tsp black pepper

Greek Yogurt Dip:
- 1 cup plain Greek yogurt
- 1 tbsp lemon juice
- 1 tsp dried dill
- 1/4 tsp garlic powder
- 1/4 tsp salt

Instructions:

1. Preheat oven to 400°F (200°C). Line two baking sheets with parchment paper.

2. In a large bowl, toss the zucchini slices with olive oil, garlic powder, paprika, salt, and pepper until evenly coated.

3. Arrange the zucchini slices in a single layer on the prepared baking sheets, making sure they don't overlap.

4. Bake for 12•15 minutes, flipping the slices halfway, until the edges are lightly browned and crispy.

5. While the zucchini chips are baking, make the Greek yogurt dip. In a small bowl, mix together the Greek yogurt, lemon juice, dried dill, garlic powder, and salt.

6. Remove the baked zucchini chips from the oven and let cool for 5 minutes.

7. Serve the warm zucchini chips with the Greek yogurt dip on the side for dipping.

Enjoy these healthy, crispy zucchini chips with the cool, tangy yogurt dip! The combination makes for a delicious and nutritious snack or appetizer.

40. Protein Shake with Banana and Almond Milk

Ingredient:

- 1 ripe banana, frozen
- 1 cup unsweetened almond milk
- 1 scoop vanilla or unflavored protein powder
- 1 tbsp almond butter (or peanut butter)
- 1 tsp honey (optional)
- 1/2 tsp vanilla extract (optional)
- Ice cubes (optional)

Instructions:

1. Add the frozen banana, almond milk, protein powder, almond butter, honey (if using), and vanilla extract (if using) to a high•powered blender.

2. Blend on high speed until the mixture is smooth and creamy, about 1•2 minutes.

3. If you want a thicker, colder shake, add a few ice cubes and blend again until the desired consistency is reached.

4. Pour the protein shake into a glass and enjoy immediately.

Tips:
- Use a ripe, frozen banana for a naturally sweet and creamy shake.
- Adjust the amount of almond milk to reach your desired thickness.
- Substitute the almond butter with peanut butter if preferred.
- Add a handful of spinach or kale for extra nutrients.
- Use a plant•based or whey•based protein powder.

This protein shake is a nutritious and delicious way to start your day or refuel after a workout. The combination of banana, almond milk, and protein powder provides a good balance of carbs, healthy fats, and protein.

41. Cucumber and Hummus Sandwiches

Ingredient:

- 1 cucumber, sliced into thin rounds
- 1 cup hummus (store•bought or homemade)
- 8 slices of whole grain bread
- Optional toppings: sprouts, sliced tomatoes, feta cheese

Instructions:

1. Slice the cucumber into thin, even rounds, about 1/4•inch thick.

2. Spread about 2•3 tablespoons of hummus evenly over 4 slices of the whole grain bread.

3. Arrange the cucumber slices in a single layer over the hummus•covered bread.

4. If using any optional toppings, layer them over the cucumber slices.

5. Top with the remaining 4 slices of bread to create 4 open•faced sandwiches.

6. Cut each sandwich in half diagonally, if desired, for easier handling.

7. Serve the cucumber and hummus sandwiches immediately.

These sandwiches make a great healthy snack or light lunch. The cool, crunchy cucumber pairs perfectly with the creamy, flavorful hummus. The whole grain bread provides complex carbs and fiber.

You can customize the recipe by using different types of hummus (e.g. roasted red pepper, garlic, or sun•dried tomato) or adding other fresh veggies like sprouts, tomatoes, or red onion. The options are endless!

42. Low•Fat Ricotta Cheese with Berries

Ingredient:

- 1 cup low•fat or non•fat ricotta cheese
- 1 cup mixed berries (such as blueberries, raspberries, blackberries)
- 1•2 tbsp honey (optional)
- Mint leaves for garnish (optional)

Instructions:

1. Scoop the ricotta cheese into a serving bowl or individual bowls.

2. Top the ricotta with the mixed berries, arranging them in a decorative pattern if desired.

3. If you want to add a touch of sweetness, drizzle 1•2 tablespoons of honey over the top of the berries and ricotta.

4. Garnish with a few fresh mint leaves, if desired.

5. Serve immediately or refrigerate until ready to enjoy.

That's it! This makes for a simple, healthy, and delicious snack or light dessert.

The key benefits of this recipe:

- Ricotta cheese is high in protein and calcium.
- Berries are packed with antioxidants, fiber, and vitamins.
- Honey provides natural sweetness (optional).
- It's a quick and easy way to enjoy a nutritious treat.

You can experiment with different types of berries or even try other fresh fruit like sliced peaches or kiwi. The ricotta and fruit combination is very versatile. Adjust the amount of honey to your personal taste preferences.

43. Sliced Turkey and Avocado Roll•Ups

Ingredient:

- 6•8 slices of deli turkey
- 1 ripe avocado, sliced
- 1 tbsp olive oil
- 1 tbsp lemon juice
- Salt and pepper to taste

Instructions:

1. In a small bowl, mix together the olive oil and lemon juice. This will be the dressing for the roll•ups.

2. Lay the turkey slices out flat on a clean surface.

3. Place a few slices of avocado near the edge of each turkey slice.

4. Carefully roll up the turkey slice around the avocado, securing it with a toothpick if needed.

5. Drizzle the olive oil and lemon dressing over the rolled up turkey and avocado.

6. Season with a pinch of salt and pepper.

7. Serve the turkey and avocado roll•ups immediately, or refrigerate until ready to serve.

These roll•ups make a great healthy snack or light lunch. The creamy avocado pairs perfectly with the savory turkey, and the lemon•olive oil dressing adds a nice bright flavor.

You can customize the recipe by using different types of deli meat, adding a slice of cheese, or using different seasonings. Just be sure to adjust the amounts of the dressing ingredients accordingly.

Enjoy these simple yet delicious turkey and avocado roll•ups!

44. Low•Fat Greek Yogurt with Honey

Ingredient:

- 1 cup low•fat or non•fat Greek yogurt
- 1•2 tbsp honey
- Optional toppings: fresh fruit, granola, nuts, cinnamon

Instructions:

1. Scoop the Greek yogurt into a bowl or serving dish.

2. Drizzle the honey over the top of the yogurt. Start with 1 tablespoon and add more to taste, if desired.

3. If using any optional toppings, sprinkle them over the honey•sweetened yogurt.

4. Serve immediately or refrigerate until ready to enjoy.

That's it! This makes for a quick, healthy, and delicious snack or breakfast.

The key benefits of this recipe:

- Greek yogurt is high in protein and probiotics, which are great for gut health.
- Honey provides natural sweetness and antioxidants.
- The toppings add extra nutrients, texture, and flavor.

Feel free to adjust the amount of honey to your personal taste preferences. Some people like their yogurt a little sweeter, while others prefer it more tart. You can also experiment with different fruit, nut, and spice toppings.

45. Veggie and Hummus Wraps

Ingredient:

- 4 whole wheat tortillas or wraps
- 1 cup hummus (store•bought or homemade)
- 1 cup shredded carrots
- 1 cup thinly sliced cucumber
- 1 cup baby spinach or arugula
- 1/4 cup crumbled feta cheese (optional)

Instructions:

1. Spread about 1/4 cup of hummus evenly over each whole wheat tortilla or wrap, leaving a small border around the edges.

2. Arrange the shredded carrots, sliced cucumber, and baby spinach or arugula in a line down the center of each tortilla.

3. If using, sprinkle the crumbled feta cheese over the vegetables.

4. Fold the bottom of the tortilla up over the filling, then fold in the sides and continue rolling it up tightly into a wrap.

5. Slice the wraps in half diagonally, if desired, and serve.

That's it! These veggie and hummus wraps make a great healthy and portable lunch or snack.

The key benefits of this recipe:

- Whole wheat tortillas provide complex carbs and fiber.
- Hummus is a good source of plant•based protein and healthy fats.
- Vegetables like carrots, cucumbers, and greens add vitamins, minerals, and antioxidants.
- Feta cheese adds a tangy, creamy element (optional).

You can customize these wraps by using different types of vegetables, swapping the hummus for another spread like avocado or tzatziki, or adding other toppings like roasted red peppers or olives.

These wraps are easy to make ahead of time and pack for work or school. Enjoy this nutritious and delicious handheld meal!

46. Baked Kale Chips with Nutritional Yeast

Ingredient:

- 1 bunch of kale, washed and dried thoroughly
- 1•2 tbsp olive oil
- 2•3 tbsp nutritional yeast
- 1/2 tsp garlic powder (optional)
- 1/4 tsp salt

Instructions:

1. Preheat your oven to 325°F (165°C). Line a large baking sheet with parchment paper.

2. Wash the kale and pat it completely dry with paper towels or a clean kitchen towel. Tear or cut the kale leaves into bite•sized pieces, discarding any tough stems.

3. Place the kale pieces in a large bowl. Drizzle with the olive oil and toss to coat the kale evenly.

4. Sprinkle the nutritional yeast, garlic powder (if using), and salt over the kale. Toss again to distribute the seasonings.

5. Arrange the kale pieces in a single layer on the prepared baking sheet, making sure they don't overlap.

6. Bake for 12•15 minutes, flipping the kale halfway through, until the chips are crispy and lightly browned.

7. Remove the baked kale chips from the oven and let them cool for a few minutes before serving.

Enjoy these crispy, flavorful kale chips as a healthy snack or side dish. The nutritional yeast adds a savory, cheese•like flavor, while the garlic powder and salt enhance the overall taste.

You can experiment with different seasonings, such as cayenne pepper, paprika, or lemon zest, to customize the flavor profile. Just be sure to adjust the amounts to your personal taste preferences.

47. Chickpea Salad with Cucumber and Tomato

Ingredient:

- 1 (15 oz) can chickpeas, drained and rinsed
- 1 cup diced cucumber
- 1 cup diced tomatoes
- 2 tbsp finely chopped red onion
- 2 tbsp chopped fresh parsley
- 2 tbsp olive oil
- 1 tbsp lemon juice
- 1 tsp Dijon mustard
- 1/4 tsp salt
- 1/4 tsp black pepper

Instructions:

1. In a large bowl, combine the drained and rinsed chickpeas, diced cucumber, diced tomatoes, chopped red onion, and chopped parsley. Mix well.

2. In a small bowl, whisk together the olive oil, lemon juice, Dijon mustard, salt, and black pepper to make the dressing.

3. Pour the dressing over the chickpea salad and toss gently to coat everything evenly.

4. Refrigerate the chickpea salad for at least 30 minutes to allow the flavors to meld.

5. Serve chilled or at room temperature. This salad can be enjoyed on its own or scooped up with whole grain crackers or pita bread.

The key benefits of this recipe:

- Chickpeas are a great source of plant•based protein and fiber.
- Cucumbers and tomatoes provide vitamins, minerals, and hydration.
- The lemon juice and Dijon dressing adds a bright, tangy flavor.
- It's a refreshing, nutritious, and easy•to•make salad.

You can customize this recipe by adding other vegetables like bell peppers, celery, or olives. You can also experiment with different herbs or spices in the dressing.

This chickpea salad makes a great healthy lunch or light dinner. Enjoy!

48. Protein•Packed Trail Mix

Ingredient:

- 1 cup raw almonds
- 1/2 cup raw cashews
- 1/2 cup raw pumpkin seeds
- 1/2 cup raw sunflower seeds
- 1/2 cup unsweetened shredded coconut
- 1/4 cup dried cranberries
- 2 tbsp chia seeds
- 2 tbsp hemp seeds
- 1 scoop (about 30g) vanilla or chocolate protein powder

Instructions:

1. In a large bowl, combine the almonds, cashews, pumpkin seeds, sunflower seeds, shredded coconut, dried cranberries, chia seeds, and hemp seeds. Mix well.

2. Add the protein powder and stir until the powder is evenly distributed throughout the trail mix.

3. Transfer the protein•packed trail mix to an airtight container or resealable bag.

That's it! This makes a nutritious and satisfying snack that you can enjoy on the go.

The key benefits of this recipe:

- Nuts and seeds provide healthy fats, protein, and fiber.
- Dried cranberries add a touch of natural sweetness.
- Chia and hemp seeds boost the nutrient content.
- Protein powder increases the protein content, making it more filling.

You can customize this trail mix by using different types of nuts, seeds, and dried fruits. Just be sure to keep the overall proportions similar.

Store the trail mix in an airtight container at room temperature for up to 2 weeks. It makes a great snack to have on hand for a quick energy boost or to take with you on hikes, road trips, or to the gym.

Enjoy this protein•packed and nutritious trail mix!

49. Cottage Cheese with Mango Chunks

Ingredient:

- 1 cup low•fat or non•fat cottage cheese
- 1 cup diced fresh mango
- 1 tsp honey (optional)
- Mint leaves for garnish (optional)

Instructions:

1. Scoop the cottage cheese into a serving bowl or individual bowls.

2. Top the cottage cheese with the diced mango chunks.

3. If desired, drizzle 1 teaspoon of honey over the top of the cottage cheese and mango.

4. Garnish with a few fresh mint leaves, if you have them on hand.

That's it! This makes for a simple, healthy, and delicious snack or light breakfast.

The key benefits of this recipe:

- Cottage cheese is high in protein and calcium.
- Mangoes are a great source of vitamins, minerals, and fiber.
- Honey provides a touch of natural sweetness (optional).
- It's a quick and easy way to enjoy a nutritious treat.

You can use any type of fresh, ripe mango for this recipe. Diced pineapple or berries would also work well as an alternative fruit topping.

Feel free to adjust the amounts of cottage cheese and mango to your personal taste preferences. Some people may prefer a higher ratio of fruit to cottage cheese.

This cottage cheese and mango combination makes for a refreshing, flavorful, and satisfying snack. Enjoy!

50. Hard•Boiled Eggs with a Dash of Salt

Ingredient:

• 6 large eggs
• 1/4 tsp salt (or to taste)

Instructions:

1. Place the eggs in a single layer in a saucepan and cover with cold water by 1 inch.

2. Bring the water to a boil over high heat. Once the water reaches a rolling boil, remove the pan from the heat and cover with a lid.

3. Let the eggs sit in the hot water for 12 minutes for hard•boiled eggs.

4. Drain the hot water and cover the eggs with cold water to stop the cooking. Let them sit in the cold water for 5 minutes.

5. Peel the eggs and place them in a serving dish or plate.

6. Sprinkle a small amount of salt, about 1/4 teaspoon, over the hard•boiled eggs.

That's it! You now have perfectly cooked hard•boiled eggs seasoned with a dash of salt.

The key benefits of this recipe:

• Hard•boiled eggs are an excellent source of protein, vitamins, and minerals.
• Salt enhances the natural flavor of the eggs.
• It's a simple, nutritious snack that's easy to prepare.

You can adjust the amount of salt to your personal taste preferences. Some people like their hard•boiled eggs more heavily salted, while others prefer a lighter touch.

Hard•boiled eggs are a versatile ingredient that can be enjoyed on their own as a snack, added to salads, or used in various recipes. Enjoy!

51. Greek Yogurt with Almonds and Honey

Ingredient:

- 1 cup plain Greek yogurt
- 2 tbsp sliced or slivered almonds
- 1•2 tbsp honey

Instructions:

1. Scoop the Greek yogurt into a bowl or individual serving dish.

2. Sprinkle the sliced or slivered almonds over the top of the yogurt.

3. Drizzle 1•2 tablespoons of honey over the almonds and yogurt, to taste.

That's it! This makes for a simple, healthy, and delicious snack or light breakfast.

The key benefits of this recipe:

- Greek yogurt is high in protein and probiotics.
- Almonds provide healthy fats, protein, and fiber.
- Honey adds natural sweetness.

You can adjust the amounts of each ingredient to your personal preference. Some people may want more or less honey, for example.

For extra flavor and texture, you can also try adding:
- A sprinkle of cinnamon
- A handful of fresh berries
- A drizzle of nut butter
- A sprinkle of granola or crushed nuts

This Greek yogurt, almond, and honey combination makes for a satisfying and nutritious snack that can help keep you feeling full and energized. Enjoy!

52. Mini Quesadillas with Chicken and Cheese

Ingredient:

- 8 small whole wheat tortillas (or 4 regular•sized tortillas, cut in half)
- 1 cup shredded cooked chicken breast
- 1 cup shredded low•fat cheddar or Monterey Jack cheese
- 1 tbsp olive oil
- Salsa, guacamole, or Greek yogurt for serving (optional)

Instructions:

1. Preheat a large skillet or griddle over medium heat.

2. Place 4 of the tortillas on a clean work surface. Evenly distribute the shredded chicken and cheese over the tortillas, leaving a small border around the edges.

3. Top each filled tortilla with another tortilla to create 4 mini quesadillas.

4. Brush the top tortillas lightly with olive oil.

5. Place the mini quesadillas, oil•side down, in the preheated skillet or griddle. Cook for 2•3 minutes per side, until the tortillas are lightly golden brown and the cheese is melted.

6. Remove the cooked quesadillas from the heat and cut each one in half to create 8 mini quesadilla triangles.

7. Serve the mini quesadillas warm, with salsa, guacamole, or Greek yogurt for dipping, if desired.

These mini quesadillas make a great healthy snack or light meal. The combination of whole wheat tortillas, lean chicken, and melted cheese provides a balance of complex carbs, protein, and healthy fats.

You can customize the fillings by using different types of cheese, adding sautéed veggies, or using shredded turkey or beef instead of chicken.

Enjoy these easy and delicious mini quesadillas!

53. Edamame with Sea Salt

Ingredient:

- 1 lb fresh edamame in the pod
- 1•2 tsp coarse sea salt

Instructions:

1. Bring a large pot of salted water to a boil.

2. Add the edamame pods to the boiling water and cook for 5•7 minutes, until the pods are bright green and tender.

3. Drain the cooked edamame in a colander and rinse with cold water to stop the cooking.

4. Pat the edamame pods dry with paper towels or a clean kitchen towel.

5. Transfer the edamame to a serving bowl and sprinkle 1•2 teaspoons of coarse sea salt over the top, to taste.

6. Serve the salted edamame warm or at room temperature.

To eat, simply pick up an edamame pod, place it in your mouth, and use your teeth to gently squeeze the beans out of the pod.

The key benefits of this recipe:

- Edamame is a great source of plant•based protein, fiber, and nutrients.
- Sea salt provides a simple, flavorful seasoning.
- It's a quick, easy, and healthy snack or appetizer.

You can adjust the amount of salt to your personal preference. Some people like their edamame more heavily salted, while others prefer a lighter touch.

Enjoy these tasty, nutritious edamame as a quick and satisfying snack!

54. Cucumber Slices with Turkey and Cheese

Ingredient:

- 1 medium cucumber, sliced into rounds
- 8•10 slices of deli turkey
- 4•6 slices of low•fat cheddar or Swiss cheese
- Optional: Dijon mustard, black pepper

Instructions:

1. Wash the cucumber and slice it into thin, even rounds, about 1/4•inch thick.

2. Lay the cucumber slices out on a plate or platter.

3. Fold or roll up the deli turkey slices and place one on top of each cucumber round.

4. Top each turkey•topped cucumber slice with a small piece of cheese, cutting the cheese slices to fit if needed.

5. If desired, you can add a small dab of Dijon mustard on top of the cheese and a light sprinkle of black pepper.

That's it! These cucumber slices with turkey and cheese make for a simple, healthy, and tasty snack or appetizer.

The key benefits of this recipe:

- Cucumbers are hydrating and provide fiber and vitamins.
- Turkey is a lean protein source.
- Cheese adds calcium and healthy fats.
- The combination of flavors and textures is really satisfying.

You can customize this recipe by using different types of deli meat (such as ham or roast beef) or cheese (like pepper jack or provolone). You can also experiment with other condiments or seasonings.

These cucumber bites are easy to assemble and make a great option for a quick, nutritious snack or a fun party appetizer. Enjoy!

55. Protein Ice Cream with Protein Powder and Almond Milk

Ingredient:

- 1 cup unsweetened almond milk
- 1 scoop (about 30g) vanilla or chocolate protein powder
- 1 frozen banana, sliced
- 1 tbsp peanut butter (optional)

Instructions:

1. In a blender, combine the almond milk and protein powder. Blend until smooth and well incorporated.

2. Add the frozen banana slices and peanut butter (if using) to the blender.

3. Blend on high speed until the mixture is thick and creamy, like soft•serve ice cream, about 1•2 minutes.

4. Serve the protein ice cream immediately, or transfer it to a freezer•safe container and freeze for 30•60 minutes for a firmer texture.

That's it! This protein•packed ice cream is a delicious and healthy treat.

The key benefits of this recipe:

- Almond milk provides a creamy base without the fat and calories of regular dairy.
- Protein powder boosts the protein content to help keep you feeling full and satisfied.
- Frozen banana adds natural sweetness and a creamy texture.
- Peanut butter provides healthy fats and extra flavor (optional).

You can customize this recipe by using different types of protein powder (e.g. chocolate, strawberry) or nut butters. You can also experiment with adding other frozen fruits like berries or mango.

This protein ice cream is a great option for a post•workout snack, a healthy dessert, or anytime you're craving something sweet and creamy. Enjoy!

56. Peanut Butter and Celery Sticks

Ingredient:

- 2•3 celery stalks, cut into 4•inch sticks
- 2•3 tablespoons creamy peanut butter

Instructions:

1. Wash the celery stalks and cut them into 4•inch sticks.

2. Spread about 1•2 teaspoons of peanut butter onto the end of each celery stick.

3. Arrange the peanut butter•topped celery sticks on a plate or platter.

That's it! This makes for a simple, healthy, and delicious snack.

The key benefits of this recipe:

- Celery provides fiber, vitamins, and minerals.
- Peanut butter is a good source of protein and healthy fats.
- It's a quick and easy snack that's satisfying and nutritious.

You can use any type of peanut butter you prefer, such as creamy, crunchy, or even almond butter or cashew butter. Adjust the amount of peanut butter to your personal taste preferences.

For added flavor, you can also sprinkle a pinch of cinnamon or a drizzle of honey over the peanut butter.

This peanut butter and celery stick combination makes a great snack on its own or can be paired with other healthy items like apple slices or whole grain crackers.

Enjoy this simple yet satisfying and nutritious snack!

57. Sliced Pears with Cottage Cheese

Ingredient:

- 1 ripe pear, cored and sliced
- 1/2 cup low•fat or non•fat cottage cheese
- 1 tbsp chopped walnuts (optional)
- 1 tsp honey (optional)

Instructions:

1. Wash and core the pear, then slice it into thin, even pieces.

2. Scoop the cottage cheese into a small bowl or plate.

3. Arrange the sliced pear pieces around the cottage cheese.

4. If desired, sprinkle the chopped walnuts over the top of the cottage cheese and pear slices.

5. Drizzle a small amount of honey over the top, about 1 teaspoon, if you want to add a touch of sweetness.

That's it! This makes for a simple, healthy, and delicious snack or light dessert.

The key benefits of this recipe:

- Pears are a good source of fiber, vitamins, and antioxidants.
- Cottage cheese is high in protein and calcium.
- Walnuts provide healthy fats and crunch (optional).
- Honey adds natural sweetness (optional).

You can use any variety of ripe pear for this recipe, such as Bartlett, Bosc, or Anjou. Feel free to adjust the amounts of cottage cheese, walnuts, and honey to your personal taste preferences.

This combination of creamy cottage cheese, sweet pear slices, and optional crunchy walnuts and honey makes for a satisfying and nutritious snack or light meal.

58. Protein•Packed Deviled Eggs

Ingredient:

- 6 hard•boiled eggs
- 2 tbsp plain Greek yogurt
- 1 tbsp Dijon mustard
- 1 tsp lemon juice
- 1/4 tsp salt
- 1/8 tsp black pepper
- 1 tbsp chopped chives (optional)

Instructions:

1. Peel the hard•boiled eggs and cut them in half lengthwise.

2. Carefully scoop the yolks out of the egg whites and place them in a small bowl.

3. Add the Greek yogurt, Dijon mustard, lemon juice, salt, and black pepper to the bowl with the egg yolks. Mash and mix everything together until smooth and creamy.

4. Spoon or pipe the yolk mixture back into the hollowed•out egg white halves.

5. Sprinkle the chopped chives over the top of the deviled eggs, if using.

6. Refrigerate the deviled eggs until ready to serve.

These protein•packed deviled eggs make a great healthy snack or appetizer. The key benefits include:

- Hard•boiled eggs are an excellent source of protein.
- Greek yogurt adds extra protein and creaminess.
- Dijon mustard and lemon juice provide a tangy flavor.
- Chives add a fresh, herbal note (optional).

You can customize the recipe by using different seasonings, such as paprika, cayenne pepper, or dill. You can also top the deviled eggs with crumbled bacon, chopped olives, or a sprinkle of smoked paprika.

These deviled eggs are a nutritious and satisfying option for a quick snack or to serve at gatherings. Enjoy!

59. Roasted Pumpkin Seeds

Ingredient:

- 1 cup raw pumpkin seeds (also called pepitas)
- 1 tbsp olive oil
- 1 tsp salt (or to taste)
- Optional seasonings: garlic powder, onion powder, chili powder, cumin, etc.

Instructions:

1. Preheat your oven to 325°F (165°C). Line a baking sheet with parchment paper.

2. Rinse the pumpkin seeds under cold water to remove any pulp or strings. Pat them dry thoroughly with paper towels.

3. In a small bowl, toss the clean, dry pumpkin seeds with the olive oil and salt until the seeds are evenly coated.

4. Spread the seasoned pumpkin seeds in a single layer on the prepared baking sheet.

5. Roast the pumpkin seeds for 18•22 minutes, stirring halfway, until they are lightly golden brown and crispy.

6. Remove the roasted pumpkin seeds from the oven and let them cool for a few minutes before serving.

7. If using any additional seasonings, sprinkle them over the roasted seeds and toss to coat.

These roasted pumpkin seeds make a delicious and nutritious snack. The key benefits include:

- Pumpkin seeds are a good source of protein, healthy fats, fiber, and various vitamins and minerals.
- Roasting brings out their nutty, toasted flavor.
- You can customize the seasoning to your taste preferences.

Store the roasted pumpkin seeds in an airtight container at room temperature for up to 1 week.

Enjoy these crunchy, flavorful pumpkin seeds as a healthy snack on their own or sprinkled over salads, yogurt, or oatmeal. They're also a great addition to trail mixes and granola.

60. Greek Yogurt with a Sprinkle of Chia Seeds

Ingredient:

- 1 cup plain Greek yogurt
- 1•2 tsp chia seeds
- Optional toppings: honey, fresh fruit, granola

Instructions:

1. Scoop the Greek yogurt into a bowl or serving dish.

2. Sprinkle 1•2 teaspoons of chia seeds over the top of the yogurt.

3. If desired, you can drizzle a small amount of honey over the chia seeds and yogurt for added sweetness.

4. You can also top the yogurt with fresh fruit, such as berries or sliced kiwi, or a sprinkle of granola for extra texture and flavor.

That's it! This makes a simple, healthy, and delicious snack or breakfast.

The key benefits of this recipe:

- Greek yogurt is high in protein and probiotics.
- Chia seeds are a great source of fiber, protein, and omega•3 fatty acids.
- Honey, fruit, and granola can provide additional nutrients and natural sweetness (optional).

You can adjust the amounts of chia seeds and any other toppings to your personal taste preferences. Some people may want more or less chia seeds, for example.

This Greek yogurt and chia seed combination is a great way to enjoy a nutritious and satisfying snack. It's also easy to prepare and can be enjoyed on its own or as part of a larger meal.

Enjoy this simple yet delicious and healthy treat!

61. Baked Sweet Potato Fries

Ingredient:

- 2 medium sweet potatoes, peeled and cut into 1/2•inch thick fry shapes
- 1 tbsp olive oil
- 1 tsp paprika
- 1/2 tsp garlic powder
- 1/2 tsp salt
- 1/4 tsp black pepper

Instructions:

1. Preheat your oven to 400°F (200°C). Line a large baking sheet with parchment paper.

2. In a large bowl, toss the sweet potato fry shapes with the olive oil, paprika, garlic powder, salt, and black pepper until evenly coated.

3. Spread the seasoned sweet potato fries in a single layer on the prepared baking sheet, making sure they don't overlap.

4. Bake for 20•25 minutes, flipping the fries halfway through, until they are tender and lightly browned.

5. Remove the baked sweet potato fries from the oven and let them cool for a few minutes before serving.

Serve the baked sweet potato fries warm, either on their own or with your favorite dipping sauce, such as ranch, honey mustard, or ketchup.

The key benefits of this recipe:

- Sweet potatoes are a great source of vitamins, minerals, and fiber.
- Baking the fries instead of frying makes them a healthier option.
- The seasoning blend adds flavor without a lot of extra calories or fat.

You can customize the seasoning by using different spices, such as chili powder, cumin, or cayenne pepper, to adjust the flavor profile.

These baked sweet potato fries make a delicious and nutritious side dish or snack. Enjoy!

62. Protein•Packed Oatmeal with Almonds

Ingredient:

- 1 cup old•fashioned oats
- 1 cup unsweetened almond milk (or milk of your choice)
- 1 scoop vanilla protein powder
- 1 tablespoon almond butter
- 1 tablespoon chopped almonds
- 1 teaspoon honey (optional)
- Pinch of cinnamon

Instructions:

1. In a small saucepan, combine the oats and almond milk. Bring to a simmer over medium heat, stirring occasionally, until the oats are cooked through and the mixture has thickened, about 5•7 minutes.

2. Remove the oatmeal from heat and stir in the protein powder until well combined.

3. Top the oatmeal with the almond butter, chopped almonds, honey (if using), and a sprinkle of cinnamon.

4. Serve hot and enjoy your protein•packed breakfast!

The combination of the oats, protein powder, almond butter, and almonds makes this a filling and nutritious breakfast that will keep you satisfied until lunchtime. Feel free to adjust the amounts of any ingredients to suit your taste preferences.

63. Cottage Cheese with Fresh Raspberries

Ingredient:

- 1 cup low•fat or non•fat cottage cheese
- 1 cup fresh raspberries
- 1•2 tsp honey (optional)

Instructions:

1. Scoop the cottage cheese into a bowl or serving dish.

2. Gently fold the fresh raspberries into the cottage cheese, taking care not to crush the berries.

3. If desired, drizzle 1•2 teaspoons of honey over the top of the cottage cheese and raspberries.

That's it! This makes a simple, healthy, and delicious snack or light breakfast.

The key benefits of this recipe:

- Cottage cheese is high in protein and calcium.
- Raspberries are packed with antioxidants, fiber, and vitamins.
- Honey provides a touch of natural sweetness (optional).

The combination of the creamy cottage cheese and the sweet, tart raspberries creates a really nice flavor and texture contrast.

You can adjust the amounts of cottage cheese and raspberries to your personal taste preferences. Some people may want more or less of each ingredient.

This cottage cheese and raspberry dish is a great way to enjoy a nutritious and satisfying snack. It's also easy to prepare and can be enjoyed on its own or with a sprinkle of granola or a drizzle of nut butter.

Enjoy this simple yet delicious and healthy treat!

64. Low•Fat String Cheese with Grapes

Ingredient:

- 2•3 pieces of low•fat string cheese
- 1 cup of fresh grapes, washed

Instructions:

1. Take the low•fat string cheese and peel or pull it into long, thin strips.

2. Arrange the string cheese strips on a plate or in a small container.

3. Wash the grapes and add them to the plate or container, placing them next to the string cheese.

That's it! This makes for a simple, healthy, and portable snack.

The key benefits of this recipe:

- Low•fat string cheese is a good source of protein and calcium.
- Grapes provide natural sweetness and antioxidants.
- It's a quick and easy snack that's satisfying and nutritious.

You can use any variety of grapes you prefer, such as green, red, or black. The combination of the creamy, savory string cheese and the sweet, juicy grapes creates a nice contrast in flavors and textures.

This snack is perfect for packing in a lunchbox, keeping at your desk, or enjoying as a quick pick•me•up. It's also a great option for kids who need a healthy, protein•rich snack.

Feel free to experiment with different types of cheese, such as low•fat cheddar or mozzarella sticks, if you prefer a different flavor profile.

Enjoy this simple yet satisfying and nutritious snack!

65. Protein•Packed Brownies with Black Beans

Ingredient:

- 1 (15 oz) can black beans, drained and rinsed
- 3 large eggs
- 1/2 cup unsweetened cocoa powder
- 1/4 cup maple syrup
- 1/4 cup creamy peanut butter
- 1 teaspoon vanilla extract
- 1/4 teaspoon salt
- 1/2 cup chocolate chips (optional)

Instructions:

1. Preheat your oven to 350°F (175°C). Grease an 8x8 inch baking pan.

2. In a food processor or high•powered blender, blend the black beans, eggs, cocoa powder, maple syrup, peanut butter, vanilla, and salt until smooth and well combined.

3. Fold in the chocolate chips, if using.

4. Pour the batter into the prepared baking pan and spread it out evenly.

5. Bake for 25•30 minutes, or until a toothpick inserted in the center comes out clean.

6. Allow the brownies to cool completely before cutting into squares.

These protein•packed brownies get their extra boost of protein from the black beans. The peanut butter and chocolate chips add delicious flavor and texture. Enjoy these fudgy, guilt•free treats!

66. Hummus and Veggie Sandwich

Ingredient:

- 2 slices of whole grain bread
- 2•3 tablespoons hummus
- 1/2 cup sliced cucumber
- 1/2 cup shredded carrots
- 1/4 cup thinly sliced bell pepper
- 1/4 cup baby spinach or arugula
- Optional: 1 slice of low•fat cheese

Instructions:

1. Toast the two slices of whole grain bread.

2. Spread the hummus evenly over one slice of the toasted bread.

3. Layer the sliced cucumber, shredded carrots, sliced bell pepper, and baby spinach or arugula over the hummus.

4. If using, place the slice of cheese on top of the veggies.

5. Top with the remaining slice of toasted bread to create a sandwich.

6. Cut the sandwich in half diagonally, if desired, and serve.

This hummus and veggie sandwich makes a nutritious and filling lunch or snack. The key benefits include:

- Whole grain bread provides complex carbs and fiber.
- Hummus is a good source of plant•based protein and healthy fats.
- Vegetables like cucumbers, carrots, and greens add vitamins, minerals, and antioxidants.
- The cheese adds extra protein and calcium (optional).

You can customize this sandwich by using different types of vegetables, swapping the hummus for another spread like avocado or pesto, or adding other toppings like sprouts or sliced tomatoes.

This sandwich is easy to make and perfect for packing in a lunchbox or enjoying at home. Enjoy this nutritious and delicious veggie•packed meal!

67. Greek Yogurt with Mixed Nuts

Ingredient:

- 1 cup plain Greek yogurt
- 2 tablespoons mixed nuts (such as almonds, walnuts, pecans, cashews)
- 1 teaspoon honey (optional)
- Pinch of cinnamon (optional)

Instructions:

1. Scoop the Greek yogurt into a bowl or serving dish.

2. Sprinkle the mixed nuts over the top of the yogurt.

3. Drizzle the honey over the nuts and yogurt, if using.

4. Optionally, sprinkle a pinch of cinnamon over the top.

That's it! This simple, protein•packed snack or breakfast takes just a minute to prepare.

The Greek yogurt provides a good source of protein, while the mixed nuts add healthy fats, fiber, and additional protein. The honey adds a touch of sweetness if desired.

You can use any combination of nuts you prefer, such as almonds, walnuts, pecans, cashews, pistachios, etc. Feel free to adjust the amounts of each ingredient to suit your taste.

This makes for a satisfying and nutritious snack or light meal. Enjoy!

68. Baked Apple Slices with Cinnamon

Ingredient:

- 2 medium apples, cored and sliced into 1/4•inch thick slices
- 1 tablespoon unsalted butter, melted
- 2 tablespoons brown sugar
- 1 teaspoon ground cinnamon
- 1/4 teaspoon ground nutmeg (optional)
- Pinch of salt

Instructions:

1. Preheat your oven to 375°F (190°C). Line a baking sheet with parchment paper.

2. In a medium bowl, toss the apple slices with the melted butter until they are evenly coated.

3. In a small bowl, mix together the brown sugar, cinnamon, nutmeg (if using), and salt.

4. Sprinkle the sugar•spice mixture over the apple slices and toss gently to coat.

5. Arrange the apple slices in a single layer on the prepared baking sheet.

6. Bake for 20•25 minutes, flipping the slices halfway through, until the apples are tender and the edges are lightly browned.

7. Serve the baked apple slices warm, either on their own or with a scoop of vanilla ice cream or a drizzle of caramel sauce.

The combination of sweet, tender apples with the warm spices of cinnamon and nutmeg makes this a delightful and healthy dessert or snack. Enjoy!

69. Almond Butter on Whole Grain Crackers

Ingredient:

- 1/4 cup creamy almond butter
- 8•10 whole grain crackers (such as Triscuits or Wasa crackers)

Instructions:

1. Spread about 1•2 teaspoons of almond butter evenly over each whole grain cracker.

That's it! This makes for a quick, easy, and nutritious snack.

The benefits of this simple snack include:

- Almond butter provides healthy fats, protein, and fiber to help keep you feeling full and satisfied.
- Whole grain crackers offer complex carbohydrates, fiber, and additional nutrients.
- It's a portable, convenient snack that can be enjoyed anytime.

You can customize this snack by using different nut or seed butters, such as peanut butter, cashew butter, or sunflower seed butter. You can also top the crackers with sliced fruit, a sprinkle of cinnamon, or a drizzle of honey for added flavor.

This combination of healthy fats, protein, and complex carbs makes for a balanced and nourishing snack that can help curb hunger between meals. Enjoy!

70. Turkey and Spinach Roll•Ups

Ingredient:

- 8 oz cream cheese, softened
- 1/4 cup grated Parmesan cheese
- 1/4 cup chopped fresh spinach
- 1/4 teaspoon garlic powder
- 1/4 teaspoon dried oregano
- 1/4 teaspoon black pepper
- 8 slices deli turkey (about 8 oz)

Instructions:

1. In a medium bowl, mix together the cream cheese, Parmesan cheese, spinach, garlic powder, oregano, and black pepper until well combined.

2. Lay the turkey slices out flat on a clean work surface. Spread about 2•3 tablespoons of the cream cheese mixture evenly over each slice of turkey.

3. Carefully roll up each turkey slice tightly, starting from the short end and rolling towards the other short end.

4. Slice each rolled•up turkey slice into 1•inch pieces.

5. Arrange the roll•ups on a serving platter or plate. Refrigerate until ready to serve.

These turkey and spinach roll•ups make a great appetizer or snack. The creamy, cheesy filling pairs perfectly with the savory turkey. You can also try variations by using different types of cheese or adding other veggies to the filling. Enjoy!

71. Greek Yogurt with Pomegranate Seeds

Ingredient:

- 1 cup plain Greek yogurt
- 1/2 cup pomegranate seeds
- 1•2 tsp honey (optional)

Instructions:

1. Scoop the Greek yogurt into a bowl or serving dish.

2. Sprinkle the pomegranate seeds over the top of the yogurt.

3. If desired, drizzle 1•2 teaspoons of honey over the pomegranate seeds and yogurt.

That's it! This makes a simple, healthy, and delicious snack or light breakfast.

The key benefits of this recipe:

- Greek yogurt is high in protein and probiotics.
- Pomegranate seeds are packed with antioxidants, fiber, and vitamins.
- Honey provides a touch of natural sweetness (optional).

The combination of the creamy, tangy Greek yogurt and the sweet, crunchy pomegranate seeds creates a really nice contrast in flavors and textures.

You can adjust the amounts of each ingredient to your personal taste preferences. Some people may want more or less yogurt, pomegranate seeds, or honey.

This Greek yogurt and pomegranate seed dish is a great way to enjoy a nutritious and satisfying snack. It's also easy to prepare and can be enjoyed on its own or with a sprinkle of granola or a drizzle of nut butter.

Enjoy this simple yet delicious and healthy treat!

72. Cottage Cheese with Peach Slices

Ingredient:

- 1 cup low•fat or non•fat cottage cheese
- 1 medium peach, sliced
- 1 teaspoon honey (optional)
- Cinnamon (optional)

Instructions:

1. Scoop the cottage cheese into a bowl or serving dish.

2. Arrange the peach slices on top of the cottage cheese.

3. Drizzle the honey over the peach slices, if using.

4. Optionally, sprinkle a light dusting of cinnamon over the top.

That's it! This simple, protein•packed snack or light meal is ready to enjoy.

The benefits of this dish include:

- Cottage cheese is an excellent source of protein, calcium, and other essential nutrients.
- Peaches provide fiber, vitamins, and natural sweetness.
- The honey (if using) adds a touch of sweetness to balance the tanginess of the cottage cheese.
- Cinnamon provides a warm, comforting flavor.

This combination of creamy cottage cheese, juicy peach slices, and optional honey and cinnamon makes for a delicious and nutritious snack or breakfast. Feel free to adjust the amounts of each ingredient to suit your taste preferences.

Enjoy this simple, yet satisfying cottage cheese and peach dish!

73. Protein•Packed Smoothie with Spinach

Ingredient:

- 1 cup unsweetened almond milk (or milk of your choice)
- 1 scoop vanilla or unflavored protein powder
- 1 cup fresh spinach leaves
- 1/2 banana, frozen
- 2 tablespoons natural peanut butter (or other nut/seed butter)
- 1 teaspoon honey (optional)
- 1/2 cup ice cubes

Instructions:

1. Add all the ingredients to a high•powered blender in the order listed.

2. Blend on high speed until the mixture is smooth and creamy, about 1•2 minutes.

3. Pour the smoothie into a glass and enjoy immediately.

This protein•packed smoothie is a great way to start your day or refuel after a workout. The combination of spinach, protein powder, peanut butter, and banana provides a nutritious blend of fiber, protein, healthy fats, and carbohydrates.

The spinach adds a boost of vitamins, minerals, and antioxidants without overpowering the flavor. The peanut butter and banana give the smoothie a creamy, satisfying texture.

Feel free to adjust the amounts of any ingredients to suit your taste preferences. You can also try using different types of nut or seed butters, frozen fruit, or even a handful of oats for added fiber and nutrients.

Enjoy this nutrient•dense smoothie as a healthy snack or meal replacement!

74. Sliced Bell Peppers with Low•Fat Ranch Dip

Ingredient:

For the Dip:
- 1 cup low•fat plain Greek yogurt
- 2 tablespoons low•fat milk
- 1 teaspoon dried parsley
- 1/2 teaspoon dried dill
- 1/4 teaspoon garlic powder
- 1/4 teaspoon onion powder
- 1/4 teaspoon salt
- 1/8 teaspoon black pepper

For the Peppers:
- 2 bell peppers (any color), washed and sliced into strips

Instructions:

1. In a small bowl, whisk together all the dip ingredients until well combined. Cover and refrigerate for at least 30 minutes to allow the flavors to meld.

2. Wash the bell peppers and slice them into long, thin strips.

3. Arrange the bell pepper strips on a serving platter or plate.

4. Serve the low•fat ranch dip alongside the sliced bell peppers for dipping.

This healthy snack or appetizer is a great way to get in some extra veggies. The cool, creamy ranch dip complements the crisp, fresh bell peppers perfectly. Feel free to use any color of bell pepper you prefer.

The low•fat Greek yogurt in the dip provides protein, while the herbs and spices add lots of flavor without a lot of extra calories or fat. Enjoy!

75. Mini Turkey Meatballs

Ingredient:

- 1 lb ground turkey
- 1/2 cup breadcrumbs
- 1/4 cup grated Parmesan cheese
- 1 egg, lightly beaten
- 2 cloves garlic, minced
- 1 teaspoon dried oregano
- 1/2 teaspoon salt
- 1/4 teaspoon black pepper

Instructions:

1. Preheat your oven to 400°F (200°C). Line a baking sheet with parchment paper or a silicone baking mat.

2. In a large bowl, combine the ground turkey, breadcrumbs, Parmesan cheese, egg, garlic, oregano, salt, and pepper. Mix until all the ingredients are well incorporated.

3. Using a small cookie scoop or spoon, form the mixture into small, bite•sized meatballs, about 1•inch in diameter.

4. Arrange the meatballs in a single layer on the prepared baking sheet.

5. Bake for 15•18 minutes, or until the meatballs are cooked through and lightly browned.

6. Serve the mini turkey meatballs warm, either on their own or with your favorite dipping sauce, such as marinara, pesto, or honey mustard.

These mini turkey meatballs make a great appetizer or snack. They are packed with protein from the ground turkey and Parmesan cheese, and the breadcrumbs help keep them tender and juicy. Enjoy!

76. Protein Cookies with Oats and Chocolate Chips

Ingredient:

- 1 cup old•fashioned oats
- 1/2 cup whole wheat flour
- 1/4 cup unflavored whey protein powder
- 1/2 teaspoon baking soda
- 1/4 teaspoon salt
- 1/2 cup unsweetened applesauce
- 1/4 cup honey
- 1 egg
- 1 teaspoon vanilla extract
- 1/2 cup dark chocolate chips

Instructions:

1. Preheat your oven to 350°F (175°C). Line a baking sheet with parchment paper.

2. In a medium bowl, combine the oats, whole wheat flour, protein powder, baking soda, and salt. Stir to mix well.

3. In a separate bowl, whisk together the applesauce, honey, egg, and vanilla extract until smooth.

4. Add the wet ingredients to the dry ingredients and stir just until combined. Fold in the chocolate chips.

5. Scoop the dough by the tablespoonful onto the prepared baking sheet, spacing them about 2 inches apart.

6. Bake for 10•12 minutes, or until the cookies are lightly golden around the edges.

7. Allow the cookies to cool on the baking sheet for 5 minutes before transferring them to a wire rack to cool completely.

These protein•packed cookies are a delicious and nutritious treat. The oats, whole wheat flour, and protein powder provide a boost of fiber and protein, while the chocolate chips add a touch of sweetness. Enjoy!

77. Cucumber Boats with Hummus

Ingredient:

- 1 large cucumber
- 1 cup hummus (store•bought or homemade)
- Optional toppings: chopped cherry tomatoes, sliced olives, crumbled feta cheese, chopped fresh herbs

Instructions:

1. Wash the cucumber and slice it in half lengthwise. Using a spoon or melon baller, scoop out the seeds from the center of each cucumber half, creating a "boat" shape.

2. Spread about 2•3 tablespoons of hummus into each cucumber boat, filling the center.

3. Top the hummus•filled cucumber boats with any desired toppings, such as chopped cherry tomatoes, sliced olives, crumbled feta cheese, or chopped fresh herbs like parsley, dill, or chives.

4. Arrange the cucumber boats on a serving platter or plate and serve immediately.

These cucumber boats with hummus make a refreshing and healthy snack or appetizer. The cool, crunchy cucumber provides a nice contrast to the creamy, protein•rich hummus. The optional toppings add extra flavor and texture.

You can use any type of hummus you prefer, such as classic chickpea, roasted red pepper, or even a flavored variety like garlic or sun•dried tomato. Feel free to get creative with the toppings as well.

This simple, no•cook recipe is a great way to enjoy a nutritious and satisfying snack. Enjoy!

78. Baked Tofu Sticks with Soy Sauce

Ingredient:

- 1 block (14 oz) extra•firm tofu, drained and pressed
- 2 tablespoons low•sodium soy sauce
- 1 tablespoon olive oil
- 1 teaspoon sesame oil
- 1/2 teaspoon garlic powder
- 1/4 teaspoon ground ginger
- 1/4 teaspoon black pepper

Instructions:

1. Preheat your oven to 400°F (200°C). Line a baking sheet with parchment paper.

2. Drain the tofu and press it between two clean towels or paper towels to remove excess moisture. Cut the tofu into 1/2•inch thick sticks or cubes.

3. In a shallow bowl, whisk together the soy sauce, olive oil, sesame oil, garlic powder, ginger, and black pepper.

4. Add the tofu sticks to the soy sauce mixture and toss gently to coat them evenly.

5. Arrange the coated tofu sticks in a single layer on the prepared baking sheet.

6. Bake for 20•25 minutes, flipping the tofu sticks halfway through, until they are golden brown and crispy on the outside.

7. Serve the baked tofu sticks warm, with any remaining soy sauce mixture drizzled over the top or on the side for dipping.

These baked tofu sticks make a great protein•packed snack or side dish. The soy sauce, garlic, and ginger provide a delicious savory flavor, while the baking process gives the tofu a crispy texture. Enjoy!

79. Apple Slices with Almond Butter

Ingredient:

• 1 medium apple, cored and sliced into thin wedges
• 2•3 tablespoons creamy almond butter

Instructions:

1. Wash and core the apple. Slice it into thin wedges or slices.

2. Spread a small amount of almond butter, about 1•2 teaspoons, onto each apple slice.

That's it! This simple snack is ready to enjoy.

The benefits of this snack include:

• Apples provide fiber, vitamins, and natural sweetness.
• Almond butter offers healthy fats, protein, and a creamy texture to balance the crunch of the apple.
• It's a portable, easy•to•prepare snack that can be enjoyed anytime.

You can customize this snack in a few ways:

• Use a different type of nut or seed butter, such as peanut butter, cashew butter, or sunflower seed butter.
• Sprinkle a pinch of cinnamon over the almond butter for added flavor.
• Drizzle a small amount of honey over the almond butter for extra sweetness.

This combination of fiber•rich fruit and protein•packed nut butter makes for a satisfying and nutritious snack. Enjoy!

80. Greek Yogurt with Honey and Walnuts

Ingredient:

- 1 cup plain Greek yogurt
- 1•2 tablespoons honey
- 2 tablespoons chopped walnuts

Instructions:

1. Scoop the Greek yogurt into a bowl or serving dish.

2. Drizzle the honey over the top of the yogurt.

3. Sprinkle the chopped walnuts over the honey•drizzled yogurt.

That's it! This simple, protein•packed snack or breakfast is ready to enjoy.

The benefits of this dish include:

- Greek yogurt is an excellent source of protein, calcium, and probiotics.
- Honey provides natural sweetness and antioxidants.
- Walnuts are a great source of healthy fats, protein, fiber, and various vitamins and minerals.

The combination of creamy Greek yogurt, sweet honey, and crunchy walnuts makes for a delicious and nutritious snack or breakfast. The honey and walnuts also add a nice textural contrast to the smooth yogurt.

Feel free to adjust the amounts of honey and walnuts to suit your taste preferences. You can also try using different types of nuts, such as almonds, pecans, or pistachios.

This Greek yogurt with honey and walnuts is a simple, yet satisfying way to start your day or enjoy a healthy snack. Enjoy!

81. Turkey Jerky with Almonds

Ingredient:

- 1 lb lean ground turkey
- 2 tablespoons low•sodium soy sauce
- 1 tablespoon Worcestershire sauce
- 1 teaspoon smoked paprika
- 1/2 teaspoon garlic powder
- 1/2 teaspoon onion powder
- 1/4 teaspoon black pepper
- 1/4 cup sliced almonds

Instructions:

1. In a medium bowl, mix together the ground turkey, soy sauce, Worcestershire sauce, smoked paprika, garlic powder, onion powder, and black pepper until well combined.

2. Line a baking sheet with parchment paper or a silicone baking mat.

3. Scoop the seasoned turkey mixture onto the prepared baking sheet and spread it out into a thin, even layer.

4. Bake at 175°F (80°C) for 4•6 hours, flipping the turkey jerky halfway through, until it is completely dried and jerky•like in texture.

5. Remove the baked turkey jerky from the oven and let it cool completely.

6. Break the dried turkey jerky into bite•sized pieces and mix in the sliced almonds.

7. Store the turkey jerky with almonds in an airtight container at room temperature for up to 1 week.

This protein•packed snack combines savory turkey jerky with crunchy almonds for a satisfying and nutritious treat. The smoked paprika, garlic, and onion powder add great flavor to the turkey. Enjoy!

82. Edamame and Carrot Sticks

Ingredient:

- 1 cup frozen shelled edamame, cooked according to package instructions
- 2•3 medium carrots, peeled and cut into sticks

Instructions:

1. Cook the frozen edamame according to the package instructions, usually by boiling or steaming for 3•5 minutes. Drain and let cool slightly.

2. Peel the carrots and cut them into long, thin sticks.

3. Arrange the cooked edamame and carrot sticks on a plate or in a bowl.

That's it! This simple, nutritious snack is ready to enjoy.

The benefits of this snack include:

- Edamame provides protein, fiber, and a variety of vitamins and minerals.
- Carrots are an excellent source of beta•carotene, fiber, and other beneficial nutrients.
- The combination of crunchy carrots and protein•rich edamame makes for a satisfying and balanced snack.

You can customize this snack in a few ways:

- Try dipping the carrot sticks in a small amount of hummus or tzatziki for added flavor.
- Sprinkle a pinch of sea salt or other seasonings over the edamame, if desired.
- Add a few sliced cucumber or celery sticks for extra crunch and hydration.

This easy, no•cook snack is perfect for a quick and healthy pick•me•up. Enjoy the edamame and carrot sticks on their own or as part of a larger meal or snack plate.

83. Hummus with Sliced Radishes

Ingredient:

- 1 cup prepared hummus (store•bought or homemade)
- 1 bunch of radishes, washed and thinly sliced

Instructions:

1. Scoop the hummus into a small bowl or serving dish.

2. Arrange the sliced radishes around the edge of the hummus, creating a colorful presentation.

That's it! This simple, two•ingredient snack is ready to enjoy.

The benefits of this snack include:

- Hummus is a great source of protein, fiber, and healthy fats from the chickpeas and tahini.
- Radishes provide a crunchy texture, as well as vitamins, minerals, and antioxidants.
- The combination of the creamy hummus and the crisp, peppery radishes makes for a refreshing and satisfying snack.

You can customize this snack in a few ways:

- Try using different types of hummus, such as roasted red pepper or garlic•herb.
- Add a sprinkle of paprika, za'atar, or other spices over the hummus for extra flavor.
- Serve the hummus and radishes with whole grain crackers or pita bread for dipping.
- Garnish with chopped fresh herbs like parsley, cilantro, or chives.

This easy, protein•packed snack is perfect for a quick and healthy pick•me•up. Enjoy the hummus and radishes on their own or as part of a larger snack or meal.

84. Protein•Packed Breakfast Burrito

Ingredient:

- 1 whole wheat tortilla or wrap
- 2 eggs, scrambled
- 2 tablespoons black beans, rinsed and drained
- 2 tablespoons shredded cheddar cheese
- 1 tablespoon salsa
- 1 tablespoon diced avocado (optional)
- Salt and pepper to taste

Instructions:

1. Scramble the eggs in a small nonstick skillet over medium heat until cooked through.

2. Warm the whole wheat tortilla or wrap according to package instructions, if needed.

3. Place the scrambled eggs in the center of the tortilla. Top with the black beans, shredded cheddar cheese, salsa, and diced avocado (if using).

4. Season with salt and pepper to taste.

5. Fold the bottom of the tortilla up, then fold in the sides and roll up tightly to create a burrito.

6. Serve the breakfast burrito immediately, or wrap it in foil or parchment paper to enjoy on the go.

This protein•packed breakfast burrito is a nutritious and satisfying way to start your day. The combination of eggs, black beans, and cheese provides a good source of protein, while the whole wheat tortilla and avocado add healthy fats and fiber.

Feel free to customize the fillings to your liking, such as adding sautéed vegetables, swapping the cheese for a dairy•free alternative, or using a different type of salsa.

Enjoy this easy and portable breakfast burrito for a quick and nourishing meal!

85. Mini Greek Yogurt Parfaits

Ingredient:

- 1 cup plain Greek yogurt
- 1/2 cup fresh berries (such as blueberries, raspberries, or strawberries)
- 2 tablespoons granola
- 1 teaspoon honey (optional)

Instructions:

1. In small glasses or jars, layer the ingredients in the following order:
   - 2•3 tablespoons of Greek yogurt
   - 1•2 tablespoons of fresh berries
   - 1 tablespoon of granola
   - Repeat the layers until you reach the top of the glass/jar.

2. If desired, drizzle a small amount of honey over the top of the parfait.

3. Refrigerate the mini parfaits until ready to serve.

These mini Greek yogurt parfaits make a delicious and nutritious snack or breakfast. The benefits include:

- Greek yogurt is high in protein and calcium.
- Fresh berries provide fiber, vitamins, and antioxidants.
- Granola adds a crunchy texture and complex carbohydrates.
- Honey (if used) provides a touch of natural sweetness.

You can customize these parfaits in a few ways:

- Use different types of berries or a mix of berries.
- Substitute the granola for other crunchy toppings like chopped nuts, seeds, or toasted coconut.
- Add a sprinkle of cinnamon or vanilla extract to the yogurt layer.
- Use flavored Greek yogurt instead of plain.

These mini parfaits are easy to prepare and perfect for on•the•go snacking or a quick, healthy breakfast. Enjoy!

86. Hard•Boiled Eggs with Sriracha

Ingredient:

• 4•6 hard•boiled eggs, peeled
• 1•2 tablespoons Sriracha hot sauce (or to taste)
• Salt and pepper (optional)

Instructions:

1. Prepare the hard•boiled eggs according to your preferred method. Once cooked, peel the eggs.

2. Place the peeled hard•boiled eggs in a bowl or on a plate.

3. Drizzle the Sriracha hot sauce over the eggs, using 1•2 tablespoons depending on your desired level of spiciness.

4. Optionally, season the eggs with a pinch of salt and freshly ground black pepper.

That's it! This simple, protein•packed snack is ready to enjoy.

The benefits of this snack include:

• Hard•boiled eggs are an excellent source of high•quality protein, as well as vitamins and minerals.
• Sriracha adds a flavorful kick of heat and spice, which can help boost metabolism and curb appetite.
• This snack is easy to prepare, portable, and can be enjoyed anytime.

You can customize this snack in a few ways:

• Try using a different hot sauce, such as Frank's RedHot or Cholula, if you prefer a different flavor profile.
• Sprinkle the eggs with a dash of paprika, garlic powder, or chili powder for additional flavor.
• Serve the Sriracha•topped eggs with sliced avocado or a side of fresh vegetables for a more substantial snack.

Enjoy these protein•packed, spicy hard•boiled eggs as a quick and satisfying snack!

87. Cottage Cheese with Melon

Ingredient:

- 1 cup low•fat or non•fat cottage cheese
- 1 cup diced melon (such as cantaloupe, honeydew, or watermelon)
- 1 teaspoon honey (optional)
- Mint leaves for garnish (optional)

Instructions:

1. Scoop the cottage cheese into a bowl or serving dish.

2. Top the cottage cheese with the diced melon.

3. Drizzle the honey over the top, if using.

4. Garnish with a few fresh mint leaves, if desired.

That's it! This simple, refreshing snack or light meal is ready to enjoy.

The benefits of this dish include:

- Cottage cheese is an excellent source of protein, calcium, and other essential nutrients.
- Melon provides fiber, vitamins, and natural sweetness.
- The honey (if using) adds a touch of sweetness to balance the tanginess of the cottage cheese.
- The mint leaves (if using) provide a refreshing, aromatic element.

This combination of creamy cottage cheese, juicy melon, and optional honey and mint makes for a delicious and nutritious snack or breakfast. Feel free to use any type of melon you prefer, such as cantaloupe, honeydew, or watermelon.

Enjoy this simple, yet satisfying cottage cheese and melon dish!

88. Greek Yogurt with Granola and Honey

Ingredient:

- 1 cup plain Greek yogurt
- 1/4 cup granola
- 1•2 tablespoons honey

Instructions:

1. Scoop the Greek yogurt into a bowl or serving dish.

2. Sprinkle the granola evenly over the top of the yogurt.

3. Drizzle the honey over the granola and yogurt.

That's it! This simple, protein•packed snack or breakfast is ready to enjoy.

The benefits of this dish include:

- Greek yogurt is an excellent source of protein, calcium, and probiotics.
- Granola provides complex carbohydrates, fiber, and healthy fats.
- Honey adds a touch of natural sweetness and antioxidants.

The combination of creamy Greek yogurt, crunchy granola, and sweet honey makes for a delicious and nutritious snack or breakfast. The honey and granola also add a nice textural contrast to the smooth yogurt.

Feel free to adjust the amounts of granola and honey to suit your taste preferences. You can also try using different types of granola, such as nut•based or fruit•flavored varieties.

This Greek yogurt with granola and honey is a simple, yet satisfying way to start your day or enjoy a healthy snack. Enjoy!

89. Low•Fat String Cheese with Cherry Tomatoes

Ingredient:

• 2•3 pieces of low•fat string cheese
• 8•10 cherry tomatoes, washed and halved

Instructions:

1. Unwrap the low•fat string cheese and pull it into long, thin strips.

2. Arrange the string cheese strips on a plate or in a small bowl.

3. Place the halved cherry tomatoes around the string cheese.

That's it! This simple, protein•packed snack is ready to enjoy.

The benefits of this snack include:

• Low•fat string cheese provides a good source of protein and calcium.
• Cherry tomatoes are a great source of vitamins, minerals, and antioxidants.
• The combination of the creamy string cheese and the juicy, sweet tomatoes makes for a satisfying and balanced snack.

You can customize this snack in a few ways:

• Try using a different type of cheese, such as low•fat mozzarella or cheddar.
• Add a sprinkle of dried herbs, such as oregano or basil, over the tomatoes.
• Serve the string cheese and tomatoes with a small handful of whole grain crackers or pita chips for added crunch.
• Drizzle a small amount of balsamic glaze or olive oil over the tomatoes for extra flavor.

This easy, no•cook snack is perfect for a quick and healthy pick•me•up. Enjoy the low•fat string cheese and cherry tomatoes on their own or as part of a larger snack or meal.

90. Baked Chicken Tenders

Ingredient:

- 1 lb boneless, skinless chicken tenders
- 1/2 cup whole wheat breadcrumbs
- 2 tablespoons grated Parmesan cheese
- 1 teaspoon garlic powder
- 1/2 teaspoon paprika
- 1/4 teaspoon salt
- 1/4 teaspoon black pepper
- 1 tablespoon olive oil

Instructions:

1. Preheat your oven to 400°F (200°C). Line a baking sheet with parchment paper.

2. In a shallow bowl, combine the breadcrumbs, Parmesan cheese, garlic powder, paprika, salt, and black pepper. Mix well.

3. Drizzle the olive oil over the chicken tenders and toss to coat them evenly.

4. Working in batches, dredge the chicken tenders in the breadcrumb mixture, pressing gently to help the coating adhere.

5. Arrange the breaded chicken tenders in a single layer on the prepared baking sheet.

6. Bake for 15•18 minutes, flipping the tenders halfway through, until they are golden brown and cooked through.

7. Serve the baked chicken tenders warm, with your favorite dipping sauce on the side, such as honey mustard or barbecue sauce.

These baked chicken tenders are a healthier alternative to fried chicken, but still deliver a crispy, flavorful coating. The whole wheat breadcrumbs and Parmesan provide a nice crunch, while the garlic and paprika add delicious seasoning.

Enjoy these protein•packed chicken tenders as a snack or part of a balanced meal. They also make a great option for kids!

91. Protein•Packed Pudding with Chia Seeds

Ingredient:

- 1 cup unsweetened almond milk (or milk of your choice)
- 1/4 cup plain Greek yogurt
- 2 tablespoons chia seeds
- 1 scoop vanilla or chocolate protein powder
- 1 tablespoon honey (optional)
- 1/2 teaspoon vanilla extract

Instructions:

1. In a medium bowl, whisk together the almond milk, Greek yogurt, chia seeds, protein powder, honey (if using), and vanilla extract until well combined.

2. Cover the bowl and refrigerate the pudding for at least 2 hours, or up to 4 days, stirring occasionally, until thickened.

3. Once the pudding has reached your desired consistency, serve it chilled.

4. You can top the pudding with additional toppings, such as fresh berries, chopped nuts, or a sprinkle of cinnamon, if desired.

This protein•packed pudding is a nutritious and satisfying snack or dessert. The benefits include:

- Greek yogurt provides a boost of protein.
- Chia seeds are a great source of fiber, omega•3s, and other nutrients.
- Protein powder helps to make this a filling, protein•rich treat.
- Honey (if used) adds natural sweetness.

You can customize this recipe by using different flavors of protein powder, such as chocolate or peanut butter, or by adding other mix•ins like cocoa powder, peanut butter, or mashed banana.

This easy, no•cook pudding is perfect for meal prep or a quick, healthy snack. Enjoy!

92. Almond Butter with Celery Sticks

Ingredient:

- 2•3 tablespoons creamy almond butter
- 2•3 celery stalks, washed and cut into 4•inch sticks

Instructions:

1. Wash and cut the celery stalks into 4•inch sticks.

2. Scoop the almond butter into a small bowl or plate.

3. Dip the celery sticks into the almond butter, coating them evenly.

That's it! This simple, two•ingredient snack is ready to enjoy.

The benefits of this snack include:

- Celery provides fiber, vitamins, and minerals, while being low in calories.
- Almond butter is a great source of healthy fats, protein, and other nutrients.
- The combination of crunchy celery and creamy almond butter makes for a satisfying and nutritious snack.

You can customize this snack in a few ways:

- Try using a different nut or seed butter, such as peanut butter, cashew butter, or sunflower seed butter.
- Sprinkle a pinch of cinnamon or a drizzle of honey over the almond butter for added flavor.
- Slice the celery into smaller pieces or use carrot sticks instead.

This easy, protein•packed snack is perfect for a quick pick•me•up or as part of a balanced meal. Enjoy!

93. Turkey and Cucumber Roll•Ups

Ingredient:

- 4 slices deli turkey
- 1/2 cucumber, sliced into long, thin strips
- 2 tablespoons cream cheese, softened
- 1 teaspoon dried dill (or 1 tablespoon fresh dill, chopped)
- Salt and pepper to taste

Instructions:

1. In a small bowl, mix together the cream cheese and dried dill (or fresh dill) until well combined. Season with a pinch of salt and pepper.

2. Lay the turkey slices out flat on a clean surface. Spread about 1•2 teaspoons of the cream cheese mixture evenly over each slice of turkey.

3. Place a few strips of cucumber at the edge of each turkey slice. Carefully roll up the turkey around the cucumber, starting from the short end and rolling towards the other short end.

4. Slice each rolled•up turkey and cucumber piece into 1•inch thick pinwheels.

5. Arrange the turkey and cucumber roll•ups on a serving plate or platter. Refrigerate until ready to serve.

These turkey and cucumber roll•ups make a great protein•packed snack or appetizer. The creamy dill•flavored cream cheese pairs perfectly with the fresh cucumber and savory turkey.

You can customize these roll•ups by using different types of deli meat, such as ham or roast beef, or by adding other fresh veggies like shredded carrots or bell pepper strips.

Enjoy these easy, no•cook turkey and cucumber roll•ups as a healthy and satisfying snack or light meal option.

94. Protein Pancakes with Blueberries

Ingredient:

- 1 cup oat flour (or whole wheat flour)
- 1 scoop vanilla protein powder
- 1 teaspoon baking powder
- 1/4 teaspoon salt
- 1 egg
- 1 cup unsweetened almond milk (or milk of your choice)
- 1 tablespoon honey (optional)
- 1 cup fresh or frozen blueberries

Instructions:

1. In a medium bowl, whisk together the oat flour, protein powder, baking powder, and salt.

2. In a separate bowl, beat the egg and then stir in the almond milk and honey (if using).

3. Pour the wet ingredients into the dry ingredients and mix just until combined. Fold in the blueberries.

4. Heat a nonstick skillet or griddle over medium heat. Scoop the batter onto the hot surface, using about 1/4 cup for each pancake.

5. Cook the pancakes for 2•3 minutes per side, or until golden brown. Flip gently to avoid breaking.

6. Serve the protein pancakes warm, with additional blueberries, maple syrup, or other desired toppings.

These protein•packed pancakes are a delicious and nutritious way to start your day. The oat flour, protein powder, and eggs provide a boost of protein, while the blueberries add natural sweetness and antioxidants.

You can customize these pancakes by using different types of protein powder, swapping the blueberries for other fresh or frozen fruit, or adding a sprinkle of cinnamon or nutmeg.

Enjoy these fluffy, protein•rich pancakes as a healthy breakfast or brunch option.

95. Cottage Cheese with Sliced Kiwi

Ingredient:

• 1 cup low•fat or non•fat cottage cheese
• 1 kiwi, peeled and sliced

Instructions:

1. Scoop the cottage cheese into a bowl or serving dish.

2. Arrange the sliced kiwi on top of the cottage cheese.

That's it! This simple, protein•packed snack is ready to enjoy.

The benefits of this snack include:

• Cottage cheese is an excellent source of protein, calcium, and other essential nutrients.
• Kiwi is rich in vitamin C, fiber, and antioxidants.
• The combination of the creamy cottage cheese and the sweet, tangy kiwi makes for a refreshing and satisfying snack.

You can customize this snack in a few ways:

• Try using different types of fruit, such as berries, mango, or pineapple, instead of kiwi.
• Sprinkle a small amount of chopped nuts or granola over the top for added crunch.
• Drizzle a teaspoon of honey over the cottage cheese and fruit for extra sweetness.
• Add a sprinkle of cinnamon or a squeeze of lime juice for extra flavor.

This cottage cheese and kiwi snack is a quick, easy, and nutritious option that can be enjoyed anytime. It's a great way to incorporate more protein, fiber, and vitamins into your day.

Enjoy this simple, yet delicious cottage cheese and kiwi combination!

96. Greek Yogurt with Cacao Nibs

Ingredient:

- 1 cup plain Greek yogurt
- 2 tablespoons cacao nibs
- 1 teaspoon honey (optional)

Instructions:

1. Scoop the Greek yogurt into a bowl or serving dish.

2. Sprinkle the cacao nibs evenly over the top of the yogurt.

3. Drizzle the honey over the cacao nibs and yogurt, if using.

That's it! This simple, protein•packed snack is ready to enjoy.

The benefits of this dish include:

- Greek yogurt is an excellent source of protein, calcium, and probiotics.
- Cacao nibs are a rich source of antioxidants, fiber, and healthy fats.
- Honey (if used) adds a touch of natural sweetness.

The combination of creamy Greek yogurt, crunchy cacao nibs, and the optional honey makes for a delicious and nutritious snack. The cacao nibs provide a subtle chocolate flavor and a satisfying crunch.

You can customize this snack in a few ways:

- Try using different types of Greek yogurt, such as vanilla or fruit•flavored.
- Add a sprinkle of chopped nuts, seeds, or granola for extra texture.
- Swap the honey for a drizzle of maple syrup or a sprinkle of cinnamon.
- Mix in a small amount of unsweetened cocoa powder for an even more intense chocolate flavor.

This Greek yogurt with cacao nibs is a simple, yet satisfying way to enjoy a protein•packed snack. Enjoy it on its own or as part of a larger meal.

97. Baked Carrot Fries with Greek Yogurt Dip

Ingredient:

For the Carrot Fries:
* 3 medium carrots, peeled and cut into thin, fry•shaped strips
* 1 tablespoon olive oil
* 1/2 teaspoon garlic powder
* 1/4 teaspoon paprika
* Salt and pepper to taste

For the Greek Yogurt Dip:
* 1 cup plain Greek yogurt
* 1 tablespoon lemon juice
* 1 teaspoon dried dill
* 1/4 teaspoon garlic powder
* Salt and pepper to taste

Instructions:

1. Preheat your oven to 400°F (200°C). Line a baking sheet with parchment paper.

2. In a large bowl, toss the carrot fry strips with the olive oil, garlic powder, paprika, salt, and pepper until evenly coated.

3. Spread the seasoned carrot fries in a single layer on the prepared baking sheet.

4. Bake for 20•25 minutes, flipping the fries halfway through, until they are tender and lightly browned.

5. While the carrot fries are baking, prepare the Greek yogurt dip. In a small bowl, mix together the Greek yogurt, lemon juice, dried dill, garlic powder, salt, and pepper.

6. Serve the baked carrot fries warm, with the Greek yogurt dip on the side for dipping.

These baked carrot fries are a healthier alternative to traditional potato fries. The Greek yogurt dip provides a cool, creamy contrast to the savory, spiced carrot fries.

You can customize the seasoning on the carrot fries by using different spice blends, such as Cajun or Italian seasoning. The Greek yogurt dip can also be flavored with other herbs and spices to your liking.

Enjoy this nutritious and delicious snack or side dish!

98. Protein Bars with Oats and Honey

Ingredient:

- 1 cup old•fashioned oats
- 1/2 cup natural peanut butter (or other nut/seed butter)
- 1/4 cup honey
- 1 scoop vanilla protein powder
- 1/4 cup chopped nuts (such as almonds or walnuts)
- 2 tablespoons ground flaxseed
- 1/4 teaspoon salt

Instructions:

1. Line an 8x8 inch baking pan with parchment paper, leaving some overhang on the sides for easy removal.

2. In a large bowl, mix together the oats, peanut butter, honey, protein powder, chopped nuts, flaxseed, and salt until well combined.

3. Press the mixture firmly into the prepared baking pan, using your hands or the back of a spoon to compact it.

4. Refrigerate the bars for at least 2 hours, or until firm.

5. Once set, lift the bars out of the pan using the parchment paper overhang. Cut into 8•10 rectangular bars.

6. Store the protein bars in an airtight container in the refrigerator for up to 1 week.

These protein•packed bars are a great on•the•go snack or healthy treat. The oats, peanut butter, and protein powder provide a boost of fiber and protein, while the honey and nuts add natural sweetness and crunch.

Feel free to experiment with different nut butters, dried fruits, or seeds to customize the flavor and texture. You can also adjust the amount of honey or protein powder to suit your preferences.

Enjoy these nutritious and satisfying protein bars!

99. Peanut Butter and Banana Smoothie

Ingredient:

- 1 ripe banana, frozen
- 1/2 cup plain Greek yogurt
- 2 tbsp creamy peanut butter
- 1/2 cup milk (dairy, almond, or oat milk)
- 1 tsp honey (optional)
- 1/2 tsp vanilla extract
- Pinch of cinnamon (optional)

Instructions:

1. Add all the ingredients to a blender.

2. Blend on high speed until smooth and creamy, about 1 minute.

3. Taste and adjust sweetness if needed, adding a bit more honey if desired.

4. Pour into a glass and enjoy immediately.

Tips:
- Using a frozen banana gives the smoothie a thick, milkshake•like texture.
- You can use any type of milk you prefer.
- Add a handful of spinach or kale for extra nutrition.
- Top with crushed peanuts, granola, or a drizzle of peanut butter.

This peanut butter banana smoothie is packed with protein, healthy fats, fiber, and natural sweetness. It makes a delicious and nutritious breakfast, snack, or post•workout recovery drink. Enjoy!

100. Sliced Avocado with Cottage Cheese

Ingredient:

- 1 ripe avocado, sliced
- 1 cup low•fat or non•fat cottage cheese
- Salt and pepper to taste
- Optional toppings: chopped tomatoes, sliced radishes, chopped chives, lemon or lime wedges

Instructions:

1. Slice the avocado in half lengthwise and remove the pit. Slice each avocado half into thin slices.

2. Scoop the cottage cheese into a bowl or plate.

3. Arrange the sliced avocado on top of the cottage cheese.

4. Season with a pinch of salt and freshly ground black pepper.

5. Optionally, you can top the dish with any of the suggested toppings like chopped tomatoes, radishes, chives, or a squeeze of citrus.

That's it! This simple combination of creamy avocado and tangy cottage cheese makes for a nutritious and satisfying snack or light meal.

The healthy fats from the avocado pair perfectly with the protein•rich cottage cheese. It's a great way to get in a serving of healthy fats, fiber, and protein all in one dish.

Feel free to adjust the amounts of each ingredient to your taste. Enjoy this easy and delicious avocado and cottage cheese dish!

101. Edamame Hummus with Veggie Sticks

Ingredient:

- 1 cup shelled edamame, cooked and cooled
- 1/4 cup tahini
- 2 tbsp fresh lemon juice
- 2 tbsp water
- 1 garlic clove, minced
- 1/4 tsp ground cumin
- 1/4 tsp salt
- 2 tbsp olive oil

Veggie Sticks:
- Carrot sticks
- Cucumber slices
- Bell pepper strips
- Celery sticks

Instructions:

1. In a food processor, combine the cooked edamame, tahini, lemon juice, water, garlic, cumin, and salt. Pulse until smooth.

2. With the food processor running, slowly drizzle in the olive oil until fully incorporated and the hummus is creamy.

3. Transfer the edamame hummus to a serving bowl.

4. Arrange the veggie sticks around the hummus for dipping.

That's it! The edamame gives this hummus a vibrant green color and fresh, slightly sweet flavor. The crunchy veggie sticks are the perfect accompaniment for scooping up the creamy hummus.

Some variations:
- Add a pinch of cayenne pepper for a little kick.
- Garnish with chopped parsley or toasted sesame seeds.
- Serve with whole grain pita chips or crackers instead of veggies.

Enjoy this healthy and flavorful edamame hummus dip!

102. Greek Yogurt with a Drizzle of Maple Syrup

Ingredient:

• 1 cup plain Greek yogurt
• 1•2 tablespoons pure maple syrup

Instructions:

1. Scoop the Greek yogurt into a bowl or serving dish.

2. Drizzle the maple syrup over the top of the yogurt, using 1•2 tablespoons depending on your desired sweetness level.

That's it! This simple, protein•packed snack is ready to enjoy.

The benefits of this dish include:

• Greek yogurt is an excellent source of protein, calcium, and probiotics.
• Maple syrup provides a natural sweetener with antioxidants and minerals.
• The combination of the creamy, tangy yogurt and the sweet maple syrup makes for a delicious and satisfying snack.

You can customize this snack in a few ways:

• Try using different types of Greek yogurt, such as vanilla or fruit•flavored.
• Add a sprinkle of cinnamon, nutmeg, or a pinch of sea salt over the top.
• Mix in a tablespoon of chopped nuts, granola, or fresh fruit for extra texture and flavor.
• Swap the maple syrup for a drizzle of honey or a sprinkle of brown sugar.

This Greek yogurt with maple syrup is a simple, yet indulgent•tasting snack that can be enjoyed anytime. It's a great way to satisfy a sweet craving while also getting a boost of protein and other nutrients.

Enjoy this easy and delicious Greek yogurt treat!

103. Turkey and Spinach Pinwheels

Ingredient:

- 8 oz cream cheese, softened
- 1/4 cup grated Parmesan cheese
- 2 cups fresh spinach, chopped
- 1/4 tsp garlic powder
- 1/4 tsp dried oregano
- 1/8 tsp black pepper
- 8 slices deli turkey

Instructions:

1. In a medium bowl, mix together the softened cream cheese, Parmesan cheese, chopped spinach, garlic powder, oregano, and black pepper until well combined.

2. Lay out the turkey slices on a clean work surface. Spread the spinach•cream cheese mixture evenly over the turkey slices, leaving a 1/2 inch border.

3. Tightly roll up each turkey slice into a spiral.

4. Slice each rolled up pinwheel into 1•inch thick slices.

5. Arrange the pinwheel slices on a serving platter. Refrigerate for at least 30 minutes before serving to allow the pinwheels to firm up.

These turkey and spinach pinwheels make a great appetizer or snack. The creamy spinach filling paired with the savory turkey creates a delicious flavor combination. Enjoy!

104. Cottage Cheese with Sliced Oranges

Ingredient:

- 1 cup low•fat or non•fat cottage cheese
- 1 medium orange, peeled and sliced

Instructions:

1. Scoop the cottage cheese into a bowl.

2. Arrange the orange slices on top of the cottage cheese.

3. Optionally, you can sprinkle a little cinnamon or a drizzle of honey over the top.

That's all there is to it! The cool, creamy cottage cheese pairs wonderfully with the sweet, juicy orange slices. This makes a refreshing and nutritious snack or light breakfast.

Some variations:
- Use a different citrus fruit like grapefruit or tangerine instead of orange.
- Add a sprinkle of chopped nuts like almonds or walnuts.
- Mix in a spoonful of chia seeds or ground flaxseed for extra fiber and nutrients.

Enjoy this simple but delicious cottage cheese and orange combination!

105. Protein Cookies with Peanut Butter

Ingredient:

- 1 cup creamy peanut butter
- 1/2 cup honey
- 1 large egg
- 1 tsp vanilla extract
- 1/2 cup oat flour (or ground oats)
- 1/4 cup unflavored whey protein powder
- 1/2 tsp baking soda
- 1/4 tsp salt

Instructions:

1. Preheat your oven to 350°F (175°C). Line a baking sheet with parchment paper.

2. In a medium bowl, mix together the peanut butter, honey, egg, and vanilla until well combined.

3. In a separate bowl, whisk together the oat flour, protein powder, baking soda, and salt.

4. Gradually add the dry ingredients to the wet ingredients, mixing until a thick dough forms.

5. Scoop rounded tablespoons of the dough and place them about 2 inches apart on the prepared baking sheet.

6. Bake for 8•10 minutes, until the edges are lightly golden.

7. Allow the cookies to cool on the baking sheet for 5 minutes before transferring them to a wire rack to cool completely.

These protein•packed peanut butter cookies are a delicious and nutritious treat. The peanut butter provides healthy fats, the protein powder boosts the protein content, and the honey adds natural sweetness.

Enjoy these cookies as a post•workout snack, healthy dessert, or anytime you need an energy boost. Store them in an airtight container for up to 1 week.

106. Hard•Boiled Eggs with Avocado

Ingredient:

• 4 hard•boiled eggs, peeled
• 1 ripe avocado, halved and pitted
• Salt and pepper to taste
• Optional toppings: paprika, chili powder, chopped chives or green onions

Instructions:

1. Slice the hard•boiled eggs in half lengthwise.

2. Scoop out the avocado flesh and place it in a small bowl. Mash the avocado with a fork until it reaches your desired consistency.

3. Place the hard•boiled egg halves on a plate or platter. Top each egg half with a spoonful of the mashed avocado.

4. Season the eggs and avocado with salt and pepper to taste.

5. Optionally, you can sprinkle the eggs with a pinch of paprika, chili powder, or chopped chives/green onions for extra flavor.

That's it! This simple combination of protein•rich hard•boiled eggs and creamy, healthy avocado makes for a nutritious and satisfying snack or light meal.

The healthy fats from the avocado pair perfectly with the protein from the eggs. This dish is great for breakfast, as a post•workout snack, or anytime you need a boost of energy and nutrients.

Feel free to adjust the amounts of each ingredient to your liking. Enjoy this easy and delicious hard•boiled egg and avocado dish!

107. Greek Yogurt with Fresh Mango

Ingredient:

- 1 cup plain Greek yogurt
- 1 ripe mango, peeled and diced
- 1•2 tsp honey (optional)

Instructions:

1. Scoop the Greek yogurt into a bowl.

2. Top the yogurt with the diced fresh mango.

3. If desired, drizzle a teaspoon or two of honey over the top.

4. Gently stir to combine.

That's it! The creamy Greek yogurt pairs beautifully with the sweet, juicy mango. The honey adds a touch of sweetness if you want it. This makes a delicious and healthy breakfast, snack or light dessert. Enjoy!

108. Protein•Packed Granola with Almond Milk

Ingredient:

- 2 cups old•fashioned oats
- 1/2 cup sliced almonds
- 1/4 cup shredded unsweetened coconut
- 2 scoops vanilla protein powder
- 1/4 cup honey
- 2 tbsp coconut oil, melted
- 1 tsp vanilla extract
- 1/4 tsp salt

For serving:
- Unsweetened almond milk

Instructions:

1. Preheat your oven to 325°F (165°C). Line a baking sheet with parchment paper.

2. In a large bowl, combine the oats, almonds, coconut, and protein powder. Stir to mix well.

3. In a small bowl, whisk together the honey, melted coconut oil, vanilla extract, and salt.

4. Pour the honey mixture over the oat mixture and stir until everything is evenly coated.

5. Spread the granola mixture in an even layer on the prepared baking sheet.

6. Bake for 15•20 minutes, stirring halfway, until the granola is golden brown.

7. Allow the granola to cool completely on the baking sheet before transferring to an airtight container.

To serve, place a portion of the granola in a bowl and pour unsweetened almond milk over the top. Enjoy!

This protein•packed granola is great for breakfast, a snack, or even as a topping for yogurt. The protein powder adds an extra boost of nutrition, while the honey, coconut, and vanilla provide natural sweetness. The almond milk makes it a delicious and satisfying meal.

Store the granola in an airtight container for up to 2 weeks. Adjust the amount of protein powder or sweetener to your taste preferences.

109. Almond Butter with Sliced Pears

Ingredient:

- 2 tbsp creamy almond butter
- 1 medium pear, cored and sliced

Instructions:

1. Spread the almond butter onto a plate or small bowl.

2. Arrange the sliced pear pieces around the almond butter.

That's it! This makes a quick and easy snack or light meal.

The creamy, nutty almond butter pairs perfectly with the sweet, juicy pear slices. The combination provides a nice balance of healthy fats, protein, fiber, and natural sweetness.

You can also try these variations:

- Use crunchy almond butter instead of creamy
- Drizzle a bit of honey over the almond butter
- Sprinkle a pinch of cinnamon over the pear slices
- Add a few chopped walnuts or pecans for extra crunch
- Serve with whole grain crackers or toast for dipping

This almond butter and pear snack is a great option when you're looking for a nutritious and satisfying treat. The healthy fats and fiber will help keep you feeling full and energized.

Enjoy this simple but delicious combination of almond butter and fresh pear slices!

110. Turkey Slices with Apple Wedges

Ingredient:

- 4•6 slices of deli turkey
- 1 medium apple, cored and sliced into wedges

Instructions:

1. Arrange the turkey slices on a plate or platter.

2. Place the apple wedges around the turkey slices.

That's it! This makes a quick and easy snack or light meal.

The savory turkey pairs perfectly with the sweet, crisp apple wedges. It's a great combination of protein, fiber, and natural sweetness.

Some variations and serving suggestions:

- Use a variety of apple types like Gala, Honeycrisp, or Fuji.
- Drizzle a bit of honey over the apple wedges.
- Sprinkle a pinch of cinnamon over the apple wedges.
- Serve with whole grain crackers or a small handful of nuts for added crunch and nutrition.
- For a heartier meal, you can roll up the turkey slices with the apple wedges inside.

This turkey and apple snack is a great option when you want something healthy, satisfying, and easy to prepare. The protein from the turkey and the fiber and vitamins from the apples make it a nutritious choice.

Enjoy this simple but delicious combination of savory turkey and sweet apples!

111. Roasted Edamame with Sea Salt

Ingredient:

- 1 cup frozen shelled edamame
- 1 tablespoon olive oil
- 1/2 teaspoon sea salt

Instructions:

1. Preheat your oven to 400°F (200°C). Line a baking sheet with parchment paper.

2. In a medium bowl, toss the frozen edamame with the olive oil until the edamame is evenly coated.

3. Spread the oiled edamame in a single layer on the prepared baking sheet.

4. Roast the edamame for 12•15 minutes, stirring halfway, until lightly browned and crispy.

5. Remove the roasted edamame from the oven and immediately sprinkle with the sea salt, tossing to coat.

6. Serve the roasted edamame warm as a snack or side dish.

The benefits of this recipe include:

- Edamame is a great source of plant•based protein, fiber, and various vitamins and minerals.
- Roasting the edamame gives it a delightful crunchy texture.
- The sea salt provides a simple, yet flavorful seasoning.

This snack is easy to prepare and makes for a satisfying, protein•packed treat. The roasting process brings out the natural sweetness of the edamame, while the sea salt adds a savory balance.

You can customize this recipe by experimenting with different seasonings, such as garlic powder, chili powder, or a blend of your favorite spices.

Enjoy these roasted edamame with sea salt as a healthy, crunchy snack or side dish. They're perfect for satisfying your salty cravings in a nutritious way.

112. Greek Yogurt with Dark Chocolate Chips

Ingredient:

- 1 cup plain Greek yogurt
- 2•3 tbsp dark chocolate chips

Instructions:

1. Scoop the Greek yogurt into a bowl or serving dish.

2. Sprinkle the dark chocolate chips evenly over the top of the yogurt.

That's it! This makes a quick and easy snack or light dessert.

The creamy, tangy Greek yogurt pairs perfectly with the rich, melty dark chocolate chips. It's a great way to satisfy a sweet craving while also getting a boost of protein, calcium, and other nutrients.

Some variations and serving suggestions:

- Use a mix of dark and milk chocolate chips for a different flavor profile.
- Add a drizzle of honey or maple syrup over the top for extra sweetness.
- Sprinkle a pinch of cinnamon or a few chopped nuts over the top.
- Serve the yogurt and chocolate in a parfait glass for a more elegant presentation.
- Enjoy it as a snack on its own or with some fresh berries or sliced fruit.

This Greek yogurt and dark chocolate chip combination is a delicious and nutritious treat that can be enjoyed any time of day. The protein from the yogurt and the antioxidants from the dark chocolate make it a great choice for a healthy indulgence.

Enjoy this simple but satisfying yogurt and chocolate chip dish!

113. Baked Sweet Potato Chips

Ingredient:

- 2 medium sweet potatoes, washed and thinly sliced (about 1/8 inch thick)
- 1 tbsp olive oil
- 1/2 tsp salt
- 1/4 tsp black pepper
- Optional seasonings: paprika, garlic powder, chili powder, etc.

Instructions:

1. Preheat your oven to 375°F (190°C). Line two baking sheets with parchment paper.

2. In a large bowl, toss the sweet potato slices with the olive oil, salt, and pepper until evenly coated.

3. Arrange the sweet potato slices in a single layer on the prepared baking sheets, making sure they don't overlap.

4. Bake for 15•20 minutes, flipping the slices halfway through, until the edges are crispy and the centers are tender.

5. Remove the baked sweet potato chips from the oven and let them cool completely on the baking sheets.

6. Once cooled, you can season the chips with any additional spices or seasonings you desire, such as paprika, garlic powder, or chili powder.

Tips:
- Make sure to slice the sweet potatoes evenly to ensure even baking.
- Soak the sliced sweet potatoes in cold water for 30 minutes before baking to help remove excess starch and make them crispier.
- Bake the chips in a single layer to allow for maximum crispness.
- Store the cooled chips in an airtight container for up to 5 days.

These baked sweet potato chips make a delicious and healthy snack or side dish. The natural sweetness of the sweet potatoes paired with the crispy texture is simply irresistible. Enjoy!

114. Cottage Cheese with Pomegranate Seeds

Ingredient:

- 1 cup low•fat or non•fat cottage cheese
- 1/2 cup pomegranate seeds

Instructions:

1. Scoop the cottage cheese into a bowl or serving dish.

2. Sprinkle the pomegranate seeds evenly over the top of the cottage cheese.

That's it! This simple combination makes a delicious and nutritious snack or light breakfast.

The creamy, protein•rich cottage cheese pairs beautifully with the sweet•tart pomegranate seeds. The vibrant red pomegranate seeds also add a lovely pop of color.

Some variations and serving suggestions:

- Drizzle a teaspoon or two of honey over the top for extra sweetness.
- Sprinkle a pinch of cinnamon or a squeeze of fresh lemon juice over the dish.
- Add a handful of chopped nuts like almonds or pistachios for crunch.
- Serve the cottage cheese and pomegranate in a parfait glass for a more elegant presentation.
- Enjoy it with whole grain crackers or a slice of toasted bread on the side.

Pomegranate seeds are packed with antioxidants, fiber, and vitamins. Combining them with protein•rich cottage cheese makes for a nutrient•dense and satisfying snack or meal.

This cottage cheese and pomegranate dish is a simple but delicious way to enjoy the wonderful flavors and health benefits of pomegranate. Give it a try!

115. Protein Pancakes with Strawberries

Ingredient:

- 1 cup oat flour (or blended rolled oats)
- 1 scoop vanilla protein powder
- 1 tsp baking powder
- 1/4 tsp salt
- 1 egg
- 1 cup unsweetened almond milk
- 1 tbsp honey (optional)
- 1 cup fresh strawberries, sliced

Instructions:

1. In a medium bowl, whisk together the oat flour, protein powder, baking powder, and salt.

2. In a separate bowl, beat the egg. Then stir in the almond milk and honey (if using).

3. Pour the wet ingredients into the dry ingredients and mix just until combined (do not overmix).

4. Heat a lightly oiled non•stick skillet or griddle over medium heat.

5. Scoop about 1/4 cup of the batter onto the hot surface and cook for 2•3 minutes per side, until golden brown.

6. Top the cooked pancakes with the fresh sliced strawberries.

7. Serve the protein pancakes warm, with additional honey or maple syrup if desired.

These protein•packed pancakes are a delicious and nutritious breakfast or brunch option. The oat flour and protein powder provide complex carbs and muscle•building protein, while the fresh strawberries add natural sweetness and antioxidants.

You can use any type of protein powder you prefer, such as whey, plant•based, or collagen. Adjust the amount of honey or syrup to your taste.

Enjoy these healthy and satisfying protein pancakes with fresh strawberries!

116. Greek Yogurt with Fresh Figs

Ingredient:

- 1 cup plain Greek yogurt
- 3•4 fresh figs, sliced
- 1•2 tsp honey (optional)

Instructions:

1. Scoop the Greek yogurt into a bowl or serving dish.

2. Arrange the sliced fresh figs on top of the yogurt.

3. If desired, drizzle a teaspoon or two of honey over the top.

That's it! This makes a simple yet delicious and nutritious snack or light breakfast.

The creamy, tangy Greek yogurt pairs beautifully with the sweet, jammy fresh figs. The honey adds an extra touch of sweetness if you want it.

Some variations and serving suggestions:

- Use a flavored Greek yogurt like vanilla or honey instead of plain.
- Sprinkle a few chopped nuts like almonds or walnuts over the top.
- Add a sprinkle of cinnamon or a squeeze of lemon juice.
- Serve the yogurt and figs in a parfait glass for a more elegant presentation.
- Enjoy it with a side of whole grain toast or granola for a more filling meal.

Fresh figs are a wonderful seasonal fruit that are packed with fiber, vitamins, and antioxidants. Combining them with protein•rich Greek yogurt makes for a nourishing and satisfying snack or breakfast.

Give this simple Greek yogurt and fresh fig dish a try • it's a delicious way to enjoy the natural sweetness of figs!

117. Hard•Boiled Eggs with Everything Bagel Seasoning

Ingredient:

- 6 hard•boiled eggs, peeled
- 2 tsp everything bagel seasoning (or make your own blend)

Everything Bagel Seasoning Blend:

- 2 tbsp sesame seeds
- 1 tbsp poppy seeds
- 1 tbsp dried minced onion
- 1 tbsp dried minced garlic
- 1 tsp coarse sea salt

Instructions:

1. In a small bowl, combine all the ingredients for the everything bagel seasoning blend and stir to mix well.

2. Place the peeled hard•boiled eggs on a plate or platter.

3. Sprinkle the everything bagel seasoning evenly over the top of the eggs, making sure to coat all sides.

4. Serve the seasoned hard•boiled eggs as a snack or part of a larger meal.

That's it! The savory, crunchy everything bagel seasoning adds so much flavor to the simple hard•boiled eggs.

This makes a great high•protein snack or side dish. The eggs provide a boost of protein, while the seasoning blend adds a tasty punch of flavor.

Some variations and serving ideas:

- Slice the eggs in half before seasoning for a prettier presentation.
- Drizzle a bit of olive oil or hot sauce over the seasoned eggs.
- Serve the eggs with whole grain crackers or sliced avocado.
- Pack them for a portable, protein•rich snack on the go.

The everything bagel seasoning can be made in advance and stored in an airtight container for up to 1 month. This makes it easy to quickly season hard•boiled eggs whenever you need a nutritious snack.

118. Protein Smoothie with Peanut Butter and Banana

Ingredient:

- 1 ripe banana, frozen
- 1/2 cup unsweetened almond milk
- 2 tbsp creamy peanut butter
- 1 scoop vanilla protein powder
- 1 tbsp ground flaxseed (optional)
- 1 cup ice cubes

Instructions:

1. Add all the ingredients to a high•powered blender.

2. Blend on high speed until smooth and creamy, about 1 minute.

3. Pour the smoothie into a glass and enjoy immediately.

This protein smoothie is a delicious and nutritious way to start your day or refuel after a workout. The combination of peanut butter, banana, and protein powder provides a great balance of carbs, protein, and healthy fats.

Here are some tips and variations:

- Use a frozen banana for a thicker, milkshake•like texture.
- Swap the almond milk for regular milk, Greek yogurt, or your milk of choice.
- Add a handful of spinach or kale for extra nutrients.
- Use chocolate or peanut butter protein powder for more flavor.
- Top with a sprinkle of cinnamon, crushed peanuts, or a drizzle of honey.
- Adjust the amount of liquid to reach your desired consistency.

This peanut butter banana protein smoothie is packed with nutrients to keep you feeling full and energized. It's a great on•the•go breakfast or post•workout recovery drink.

Enjoy this delicious and healthy smoothie!

Congratulations on reaching the end of the "Snack Cookbook for Teens: Satisfy Your Snack Cravings with Fun and Easy Recipes With 115+ Recipes." By now, you've explored a wide array of snacks that are not only delicious but also fun and simple to prepare. We hope these recipes have inspired you to get creative in the kitchen and make snacking a delightful part of your day.

A New Way to Snack

You've learned that snacking can be both nutritious and enjoyable. The recipes in this book are designed to provide you with the energy and nutrients you need to power through your busy days while still treating your taste buds to exciting flavors and textures. By choosing healthy, homemade snacks, you're taking an important step towards a balanced and healthy lifestyle.

The Joy of Cooking

Cooking your own snacks is not just about eating well; it's also about enjoying the process. Experimenting with new ingredients, flavors, and techniques can be a lot of fun. We hope this cookbook has shown you that the kitchen is a place for creativity and exploration. Whether you're a seasoned cook or just starting out, there's always something new to discover.

Share the Love

Food brings people together, and snacks are no exception. Share these recipes with your friends and family, and enjoy the experience of making and eating delicious snacks together. Hosting a snack-making party or simply preparing treats for your loved ones can create lasting memories and strengthen your bonds.

Keep Snacking Smart

As you continue your snacking journey, remember the principles of balance and moderation. Incorporate a variety of snacks into your diet to ensure you're getting a wide range of nutrients. Listen to your body's hunger and fullness cues, and enjoy each snack mindfully.

Thank you for choosing the ***"Snack Cookbook for Teens."*** We hope it becomes a go-to resource for all your snacking needs. The recipes and tips provided are just the beginning —feel free to adapt and create your own snack masterpieces. Your enthusiasm for trying new things and making healthier choices is commendable, and we're excited to be a part of your journey.

www.ingramcontent.com/pod-product-compliance
Lightning Source LLC
Chambersburg PA
CBHW081549250726
48653CB00009B/3345

4. Hard•Boiled Eggs

Ingredient:

- Eggs (as many as desired)
- Water

Instructions:

1. Place the eggs in a single layer in a saucepan and cover with cold water by 1 inch.

2. Bring the water to a boil over high heat. Once the water reaches a full boil, remove the pan from the heat and cover.

3. Let the eggs sit in the hot water for the following times, depending on how you like your eggs:
- Soft•boiled: 3•5 minutes
- Hard•boiled: 12 minutes
- Extra hard•boiled: 15 minutes

4. Drain the hot water and cover the eggs with cold water. Let sit for 5 minutes to cool completely.

5. Gently tap each egg on the counter to crack the shell, then peel starting from the wider end of the egg.

6. Rinse the peeled eggs under cold water to remove any remaining shell pieces.

7. Enjoy the hard•boiled eggs as is, or use them in recipes like deviled eggs, egg salad, or as a protein•packed snack.

Tips:
- Older eggs peel more easily than very fresh eggs.
- Adding a teaspoon of baking soda to the cooking water can also help with peeling.
- Store hard•boiled eggs in the refrigerator for up to 1 week.

5. Protein Smoothie with Spinach and Berries

Ingredient:

- 1 cup unsweetened almond milk (or milk of your choice)
- 1 scoop vanilla protein powder
- 1 cup fresh spinach leaves
- 1 cup frozen mixed berries (such as blueberries, raspberries, and blackberries)
- 1 tbsp chia seeds or ground flaxseeds (optional)
- 1 tsp honey or maple syrup (optional)

Instructions:

1. Add the almond milk, protein powder, spinach, frozen berries, and chia/flax seeds (if using) to a high•powered blender.

2. Blend on high speed until the mixture is smooth and creamy, about 1•2 minutes.

3. Taste and add a teaspoon of honey or maple syrup if you'd like it a bit sweeter.

4. Pour the smoothie into a glass and enjoy immediately.

The key components:

Protein Powder:
- Choose a high•quality, plant•based or whey protein powder to boost the protein content.

Spinach:
- Spinach is packed with vitamins, minerals, and antioxidants, providing a nutritional boost.

Berries:
- Frozen berries add natural sweetness, fiber, and additional vitamins and antioxidants.

Chia/Flax Seeds (optional):
- These add healthy omega•3 fatty acids, fiber, and extra nutrition.

This smoothie is a great way to start your day or enjoy as a nutritious snack. The protein, greens, and fruit make it a well•balanced and filling option.

Feel free to experiment with different fruit and veggie combinations to find your favorite flavor profile. Enjoy!

6. Cottage Cheese with Pineapple

Ingredient:

- 1 cup low•fat or non•fat cottage cheese
- 1/2 cup diced fresh pineapple
- 1 tsp honey (optional)

Instructions:

1. In a small bowl, combine the cottage cheese and diced pineapple.

2. If desired, drizzle the honey over the top and stir gently to combine.

That's it! This healthy snack or light meal is ready to enjoy.

The key components:

Cottage Cheese:
- Cottage cheese is high in protein and low in fat, making it a nutritious choice.
- Look for low•fat or non•fat varieties to keep the calorie and fat content down.

Pineapple:
- Fresh pineapple adds a sweet, tropical flavor and a nice textural contrast to the cottage cheese.
- Pineapple is also a good source of vitamin C and other beneficial nutrients.

Honey (optional):
- A small drizzle of honey can enhance the sweetness if desired, but it's optional.

This simple combination of creamy cottage cheese and juicy pineapple makes for a refreshing and satisfying snack or light meal. It's easy to prepare and provides a nice balance of protein, carbohydrates, and natural sweetness.

You can also try adding other fresh fruit like berries, diced mango, or sliced kiwi for variety. Enjoy!

7. Edamame Pods

Ingredient:

- 1 lb fresh edamame pods
- 1•2 tbsp coarse sea salt or kosher salt

Instructions:

1. Bring a large pot of water to a boil over high heat.

2. Add the edamame pods to the boiling water and cook for 5•7 minutes, until the pods are bright green and tender.

3. Drain the edamame in a colander and immediately transfer to a bowl of ice water to stop the cooking.

4. Once cooled, drain the edamame again and pat dry with paper towels.

5. Transfer the edamame pods to a serving bowl and sprinkle generously with the coarse salt.

That's it! The edamame is now ready to enjoy.

To eat, simply pick up a pod, place it in your mouth, and use your teeth to gently squeeze the beans out of the pod. Discard the empty pod.

The key things to note:

- Fresh, unshelled edamame is the way to go for maximum flavor and texture.
- Boiling the pods briefly helps soften them and bring out their natural sweetness.
- The coarse salt adds a delicious salty contrast to the beans.

Edamame is a great source of plant•based protein, fiber, and various vitamins and minerals. It makes a healthy, satisfying snack. Enjoy!